M000311136

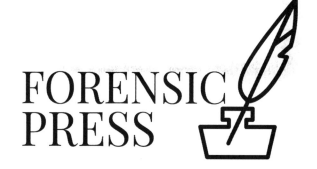

FORENSIC
PRESS

Forensic Press is an imprint of
The Forensic Criminology Institute (Sitka, Alaska)

DEAD IN IN SIX MINUTES

THE BIOGRAPHY OF DR. STANLEY M. ZYDLO JR. MD AND THE CREATION OF THE MODERN PARAMEDIC & EMS SYSTEM

PAUL CIOLINO

ISBN: 978-1-48358-508-6

"Late on the night of November 27, 1974, a skinny, 16-year-old kid chugged his hopped-up '65 Pontiac down Dundee Road in Arlington Heights. Nearby, another driver – blind-drunk – careened through Arlington Heights in his F-250 4x4 pickup. Inevitably, the truck ran a light and the two 'met' at an intersection, ricocheting the Pontiac into oncoming lanes. The kid, injured and laying on the floor of the car would eventually recover – because a man he would never meet, Stan Zydlo, had thrown his whole life into preparing for this accident, in the Northwest suburbs of Chicago.

Dr. Stanley Zydlo fought bureaucracy, entrenched policies, budgets and naiveté to create in the Chicago 'burbs, what we now know nationwide as the Paramedic system. I remember very little about that night in Arlington Heights, but I remember *"Paramedics"* prying open the door of my Pontiac and giving me aid. I had never heard of Paramedics before and I didn't know who they were or where they came from. But we all need to. And nobody can tell the story better than Paul Ciolino. If you want the real story, the unvarnished, unspun, gritty truth, this is the book you must read. Ciolino dives into this world-changing subject with gusto, and you'll feel his frustration, join in his celebration and learn of the unsung heroism of Dr. Zydlo and the people who helped him make *'Paramedic'* a household name. If you prefer the polished, politically-correct, inoffensive story of how Paramedics came to be, you're holding the wrong book. Put it down. You're wasting your time."

–Steve Moore, FBI Supervisory Special Agent, (Retired)
CNN Law Enforcement Contributor, author of, "Special Agent Man".

"Paramedics are an integral part of the fabric of society that we take for granted every day. As we go about our lives, we expect criminals to be caught, fires to be extinguished and as surely as the sun rises in the east that paramedics be poised to save lives at the sound of an alarm. <u>Dead</u> <u>in</u> <u>Six</u> <u>Minutes</u>, by Paul Ciolino, is a gritty, told-from-the-heart story of Dr. Stanley Zydlo, the Chicago physician and medical pioneer responsible for creating the system of men and women who have saved an uncountable number of lives."

– Maurice Possley, Pulitzer Prize winning journalist and New York Times best-selling author.

"<u>Dead</u> <u>in</u> <u>Six</u> <u>Minutes</u> takes you inside the lives of Paramedics on the front lines of American cities. Often taken for granted, these men and women deliver for the tax payers day after day as first responders. Paul Ciolino tells their story with candor, courage, and a lot of heart."

– Jack Murphy, Former Special Forces and Ranger, Editor-in-Chief, SOFREP.com

"Paul captures the hard work and dedication it takes to be a paramedic, performing under extreme conditions, during people's darkest moments. His background and insight into modern EMS is remarkable."

– Jeffrey A. Lyle, Deputy District Chief, Chicago Fire Department

An outstanding work of history about Dr. Stanley Zydlo MD, a major contributor to American culture. An excellent display of present day relevance that speaks to the future of medicine.

– Thomas Lee Wright Film Maker & Author

In Dead in Six Minutes, author Paul Ciolino takes us on a riveting journey across the wild frontier of urban medicine and introduces us to a true visionary who literally changed all of our lives forever. After bearing witness to a senseless tragedy, Dr. Stanley Zydlo launched himself into a desperate mission to help men, women and children at the most critical moments of their lives - the minutes and seconds that at times horrify you, make you shake with anger, but will ultimately inspire you in ways that few books can, –

– Casey Sherman, *New York Times* Bestselling Author of *The Finest Hours*

Dedicated to Joyce Reid Zydlo

Dr. Stanley M. Zydlo Jr. M.D. was simply one of those rare individuals who come along once every generation. He was a brilliant medical doctor, a humanist of the first degree, and a visionary who refused to let anyone or anything get in his way. His paramedics came to worship and respect him like very few leaders have ever experienced. His professional accomplishments are chronicled here and in numerous other media sources detailing a fifty-year career.

What was seldom mentioned in all of these outlets was how Stan was able to accomplish all of these goals and programs to a level that was legendary and unheard of. You simply do not accomplish what Dr. Zydlo accomplished in a vacuum. There are many moving parts, some more critical than others.

He never failed to brag about Joyce's beauty and dedication, as well as her accomplishments as a mother, caretaker, and other attributes. As Stan would on occasion say, "The best goddamn wife any man ever had". Stan understood the importance of Joyce's role in his life. He never failed to recognize that and he never for a second waivered in that belief.

I have been friends with Joyce for as long as I knew Stan. I have watched her handle tragedy with grace and maturity. She was Stan's rock in all of his endeavors. During the long and often bumpy journey of writing this book, especially when Stan became ill and incapacitated, and they both experienced the tragic loss of Josh, their oldest son, Joyce helped pick up the pieces so that this work could be finished. Stan was unquestionably the driving force behind the paramedics and prehospital care. Joyce was simply the support system that allowed Stan to do what he did.

All great stories have a hero who has to overcome seemingly impossible odds. There are always problems, roadblocks, and issues that seem insurmountable. In a happy ending, the hero of the story overcomes the obstacles and does what needs doing. Certainly, Dr. Zydlo did all of that. The back-story, though, is unquestionably that none of this would have been possible had Joyce Zydlo insisted on a "normal marriage and home life".

For that, and all of the above stated reasons, it is with great warmth, respect, and gratefulness that this book is dedicated to Joyce Reid Zydlo.

TABLE OF CONTENTS

INTRODUCTION

METAPHORICALLY SPEAKING, THIS BOOK IS ABOUT DAVID SLAYING GOLIATH. It's about the Great Santini. It's about King Leonidas. It's about Texas Ranger Captain Augustus "Gus" McCrae. It's about Sergeant Audie Murphy. It's about Elliot Ness. It's about General George Patton. In reality, it's about the life of Dr. Stanley M. Zydlo, Jr., MD. Zydlo was a combination of the heroic and fictionalized characters listed above. I combined fictionalized characters with real, heroic ones because Stan, at the end of the day, was as heroic and real as any of them.

He was not patient. This was not Marcus Welby, MD or Dr. Heathcliff Huxtable, or even Doug Ross from ER. He was profane. He was loud. He was edgy. He was not model good-looking. He was all sharp edges and hawkish. He suffered no fools and he cut to the chase immediately. He was in a fucking hurry and you had better get out of his way or else. This is Braveheart, or William Wallace, on steroids. It is also real life and Dr. Stanley M. Zydlo, Jr., MD, was larger than life and full of bravado. He did not have one second for political correctness, tea at noon in the doctor's lounge, or any of your bullshit.

In fact, for many years he did not have time for eating, sleeping or making love to his wife. For over ten years, he was in the middle of single-handedly changing the way we go about saving human lives. It was a long time before he had anyone else to help him.

Forty-plus years ago, if you made it to the emergency room alive, it was a miracle. Here are the simple facts. There were no 911 centers. There were no paramedics. There were no emergency medical technicians. There were no lifesaving drugs or CPR being administered to critically injured or seriously ill people. There certainly wasn't radio communication between the ER and the ambulance personnel.

For all of the brain power that has shown up at medicine's door, how is it possible that someone didn't consider these services? Well, meet Stanley Zydlo. He figured it out and absolutely changed how medicine is practiced in this country.

Everything that came afterward was based on what Zydlo had sewn together in 1972. Every Emergency Medical Service (EMS) in the country owes its beginning to Dr. Zydlo and the original ten suburban towns that agreed to participate and supply personnel and equipment. Fifteen minutes after the service went online, they saved their first life. Since that time, they have literally and collectively saved millions of lives.

Back in 1958, Stan Zydlo, a young, innocent, medical student, watched young, grammar school age children hurl themselves out of second story windows at the Our Lady of the Angels Grammar School fire on Chicago's west side. He watched fire and police personnel look on in horror. The seed was planted. On the flaming backs of those child victims, Stan Zydlo realized what had to be done.

He didn't go home or to school and write up a detailed plan, but he walked away from that tragedy with an idea. He would figure out a way to make sure that when a tragedy like this happened again, there would be trained personnel present to help. There would be ambulances that did something besides drop off bodies at morgues and funeral homes. He knew with every ounce of his being that he, Stan Zydlo, a Polish kid from the west side of Chicago, would get this shit straightened out.

A lesser man would have taken the easy way and become a dermatologist or internist. Not Zydlo. No way in hell. Even though there was not a hint of what emergency room medicine would evolve into paramedics, or emergency medical systems, Stan Zydlo did not let any of that slow him down. Out of the ashes of the Our Lady of the Angels fire, the Phoenix now known as EMS rose magically and it would save millions of lives from every corner of the world in the years to come.

So what you read here, what you learn here, you are getting from the original source(s). The acts herein are all extraordinary acts done by ordinary people. These are your neighbors, brothers, sisters, and children. None of them were born wealthy or privileged. None of them were the beneficiary of an Ivy League education. Not one of them did what they did for selfish or financial reasons.

What these men did was produce a system of medical care that should have been around for generations. It wasn't, and so they created it. People often died unnecessarily because the medical and public service entities that should have come up with this concept at least two or three generations before, did not.

Today's modern emergency room (ER) is a well-orchestrated life-saving machine. We would not change much because this is where your life gets saved in such a routine manner that it isn't even news outside of your immediate family. This is where medical miracles often take place and are so common in this country we have come to snooze through them.

This is the active combat zone of medicine. The ER docs interact with all of the drama that humans bring like combative, drug-addled patients who wake up trying to kill them. They deal with all the gunfight victims, gang riot victims, and the rest of the drama that is played out daily in our country. Yet the ER doctors are never appropriately compensated for all the talent that he or she brings to the table. They are still the redheaded stepchildren of medicine.

Historically, the paramedics and emergency medical technicians were not a new idea. The U.S military and their highly efficient combat medics had been around for at least four wars. Medics had been treating life-threatening injuries on the scene for generations. Their skills were unmatched and certainly no one ever thought it was a bad idea to have these guys around when the shit literally hit the fan and bullets started flying through the air. It's no surprise that Dr. Zydlo, Paramedic Collier, and several other originators had military backgrounds. They had seen first-hand what combat medics were capable of. Why not transfer these skills to the civilian sector? Why not, indeed?

There were some variations. There were some people who had concepts. In Seattle, WA; Ohio, California and Miami, a few people attempted to hash out something that resembled an emergency medical services system. Make no mistake about it, though, the *first*, the Granddaddy of them all was developed and created by Stan Zydlo and a few of his pals on the outskirts of Chicago in 1972.

So what took the civilian medical establishment sixty or seventy years to do what the military had been doing for damn ever? No one knows, but it looks like the same old problem: bureaucracies, politics, power struggles, money and apathy. This is why this story is so important. It is yet another example of what Americans are capable of producing when they can get away from the game playing that occurs when brilliant ideas are hatched.

This book is about remembering and giving credit to a really small circle of people who changed the face of emergency medicine. Looking back with mature reflection crystallizes their heroic and 'can do' spirit. The ability to do for others and continually go far above and beyond the call of duty was unsurpassed. They often did it while waging a war to keep doing it. Not only were their efforts often ignored, but they were accused of being thugs, gangsters, and outlaws.

What follows in these pages is the factual story of how one man literally saved millions of lives. Because of his efforts, and the fight he took on and won, just about every human in this country, and millions of others in the world, have been touched by his actions. This is a story worth telling and, I hope, worth knowing. It is one of the great stories of this nation, and it is America at its finest.

We live in a time that is unpredictable. Life moves at warp speed and there truly is no time to smell the roses. Generally speaking, the more education and brains one possesses, they are busier and the more responsibility they have. Make no mistake about it, in America, there is a societal pecking order and medical doctors are still near, or at, the head of it. Certainly, since the close of WWII, there has been a hierarchal order that the upper classes have followed. Attorneys, engineers, financial analysts and computer programmers are the career titles that a vast majority of parents and caretakers encourage their children to seek. The gold standard, however, has always been medicine.

Our best and brightest have always been encouraged to pursue a medical degree. Our society has rewarded these individuals with economic rewards often commensurate with a dozen or more years of advanced medical study. The marathonic path that doctors participate in generally rewards them with the money and prestige that we afford professional athletes or entertainers. Seven figure, annual salaries are not unheard of.

In the medical field, there is an unwritten, yet undefined order amongst the professionals. Neurosurgeons, transplant and cardiovascular surgeons are generally the rock stars of medicine. Oncologists, obstetricians, and plastic surgeons are also extremely well-compensated. Emergency room doctors are not even close in the financial arena.

Now, think about what ER doctors are required to do to be current. They have to be able to make split second decisions about administering drugs, assessing the damages, and an array of other decisions that can have a very negative affect on a patient, perhaps even kill a patient, which may cost their hospital millions of dollars. Never mind what happened prior to the patient arriving, if an ER doctor laid his hands on the patient at any juncture during the process, he or she will likely be the subject of some very serious ramifications. Working in, or running, the emergency room at a large, urban, Level One trauma center is not for the faint of heart.

There are many heroes in this story. There is Janet Schwettman, an Inverness, Illinois housewife who was a driving, unrelenting force to get the paramedic program off the ground. After being introduced to Dr. Zydlo, she never let up. She politicked, attended paramedic classes, testified at the state house, badgered politicians of both parties and begged special interest groups until they supported the law that established the paramedic program. She never quit and I don't believe she slept much during those early months. At one point, she told her husband that the only thing she wanted for Christmas was a Xerox machine. Jan died not too long ago. She was, without question, a critical cog in this process; another saint, or perhaps even more aptly called a "Guardian Angel".

There were also heroes in the politicians who got behind the paramedic bill and recognized it for what it truly was and that was a non-political act of law that saved lives. This may sound like an easy law to support, but getting behind it and passing it proved to anything but easy.

Illinois State Senator John A. Graham from Barrington, IL., was the driving force behind the bill. The historical record is quite clear. Graham was primarily responsible for writing and sponsoring the bill after Governor Richard Ogilvie recommended Graham to Mrs. Schwettman for help in getting it done. It turned out to be great advice.

Then, there were the initial classes that Dr. Zydlo instructed. Remember, this was virgin territory. The firemen who volunteered were really on thin ice, professionally. Nobody predicted that they would all become media darlings and frigging heroes. No, there was a lot of institutional resistance in the fire departments. The old school guys were dug in and unconvinced that this would benefit the fire service.

Very few of the paramedics, if any, had medical backgrounds. Education wise most were high school graduates. A few had bachelor degrees. The first chiefs, after considering it for awhile, took the plunge. Next to Dr. Zydlo and Mrs. Schwettman, the fire chiefs were absolutely heroic in their zeal to get this program up and running.

Finally, we get to the men and ladies. I apologize in advance, but the initial classes of paramedics had no women. The simple explanation is that there were no women firefighters in these particular fire departments yet. Nevertheless, Jan Schwettman and Dr. Marjorie Smith, a Northwest Community physician, who promoted and pushed the program's inception, aptly represented the female gender. The female paramedics came along after they became regular firefighters. They have, of course, served valiantly and with distinction since being allowed to participate.

There was also the long-suffering Joyce Zydlo, the doctor's wife. Without Joyce's encouragement and Stan's superhuman early efforts, the program would never have come to fruition. For ten long years, Joyce basically raised four children by herself. Dr. Zydlo gave up a very lucrative medical career, and all the perks that went with it, to guarantee excellence while training the program's paramedics. He was not compensated for those activities and, at one point, took several months off without pay to set up a training program.

It was obvious during the course of writing this book that no one, with the exception of Stan Zydlo, really knew how all of this would turn out. That is a fact and it really puts out there the genius of Zydlo. We all know that in this country where everything is pretty much driven by money, influence, and connections, there are very few things that are handled pretty much equally for everyone.

The exception is the paramedic system. When the paramedics roll, they don't consider if you have insurance. They don't care if you are wealthy or poor. They don't treat you based on where you went to college or whether your car is a Porsche or an '84 Chevy with rusted out holes in the floorboards. This is the one place where you are guaranteed to be treated the same whether you a U.S. Senator or an unemployed plumber. We owe this to Dr. Stanley M. Zydlo, Jr.

I knew Stan for over twenty years. I met him as a patient who was wheeled into his emergency room on an Easter Sunday. For all practical purposes, I was dead. He brought me back. We became friends that day. Since discovering his extraordinary history, I ragged his ass about getting his life story on paper. "Yeah, yeah, yeah. I'll get to it." But, he never got to it because he was just too humble to acknowledge his own greatness. Intellectually, he understood what he accomplished. Emotionally, though, I suspect he was just too humble to draw the attention to himself.

For a million reasons, he would never write that book. Thus, I was forced into the role of his biographer. There are probably ten thousand people more qualified to write his story. In fairness to Stan's genius, I really should not be chronicling his life. But, for a number of valid and maybe not so valid reasons here we are. I hope I did his story the justice it so richly deserved. This is Stan's life and words. I am merely the organizer of that data and information.

For over thirty years, I have been an investigator. I have worked for the state and federal governments. I have worked for myself. This has allowed me to have experiences that ordinarily would never have happened to me.

I have been absolutely blessed by the fact that my work has brought me into contact with people whose spirit and contributions to society and their fellow man have gone so far beyond what anyone would or could expect, and in reality, we should classify them as "Saintly".

I would love to hear what the naysayers and haters think now. With every ounce of their collective being, they attempted to block Stan Zydlo and his merry little band of men. They were almost successful. What they failed to take into account was the honor and valor of those who created this brand of gunslinger medicine. What they misjudged was Stan Zydlo's genius and heart. Lucky for the rest of us, they did.

CHAPTER ONE

Mr. Rogers Does Not Live Here

"The wisest are the most annoyed at the loss of time."
– Dante Alighieri

When Shakespeare wrote Henry IV, Part 1, the story of Prince Hal (the future King Henry V of England), a fifteenth century wild child who caroused with criminals and commoners, helped his loser chums rob his father's treasury and spent all his time in seedy bars, he did not realize he was writing about young Stan Zydlo.

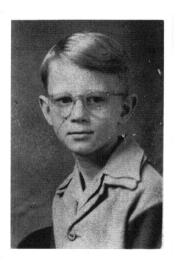

Stan Zydlo circa 1940. Courtesy Zydlo family

Zydlo, a wild child who hung out with gang members and would later hang out with commoners (firemen), grew up in a tavern on Chicago's wild, West Side. His father was "kinglike" in this realm. He was a Chicago alderman which, as anyone from Chicago knows, is very much a king in his patch of territory.

Shakespeare describes Prince Hal's story as taking place before his glorious transformation from a total disgrace into a noble leader who helped put down an uprising that threatened his father's reign, and killed the guy badmouthing his father.

Zydlo transformed himself from a street brawling tough guy into one of the most respectable medical doctors of the twenty-first century. He did all this in spite of the entire medical establishment trying to destroy him by whispering into the collective ear of the media that Zydlo's father was a former Chicago alderman who had been convicted of political corruption. Indeed, the Zydlo-Shakespeare angle is eerily familiar, in spite of having been written five hundred years apart. The vast majority of Stan's colleagues had no idea where he came from. Few knew, or cared, about his hard scrabble beginnings. Medical professionals cull the herd quickly. Just to get accepted into an American medical school is akin to winning the lottery. Once admitted, the instructors, deans and staff physicians look for any weakness. If they find it, they hack at it until you quit or they can discharge you. Most of them take great pleasure in this and no one cares one whit about a former med school student.

Stan Zydlo's ascension to medical school was, considering where he came from, a winning lottery ticket, albeit he had to perform a few super human academic feats before being admitted. The journey wound up being far more interesting than the actual arrival and completion.

S&W Tap was a typical Chicago saloon known in Chicagoese as a tavern, gin mill, or simply a "joint." Every possible human drama is played out daily in these oases of booze, and back then, cigarette smoke. This was a workingman's place. There were no dress codes. A beer could cost as little as a nickel and a shot of cheap booze, 25 to 50 cents. Usually, the owner, or a family member, was the bartender. Each tavern, and there were hundreds of them, was the cornerstone of the ethnic neighborhoods. Tabs, though illegal, were routinely given to regulars who cashed their paychecks there, for a small fee.

In Chicago, a neighborhood is a two or three block area where all the residents know one another or at least are familiar with who belongs and who doesn't. This was Stan's landscape. The smell of piss, bad booze, and dirty ashtrays was the backdrop of his childhood.

The local police came by once a week for an envelope stuffed with cash. The bookie at the end of the bar took bets twelve hours a day. The pay phone belonged to him and he never got off it. Throw in the fact that Stan's father, (Stan, Sr.) was the ward alderman and you had every resident stopping by for favors.

"Hey, Stan, can you get my kid on the fire department?"

"Hey, Stan, can you fix this parking ticket?"

"See the cop at the end of the bar."

"Stan, I need a zoning variance for my garage."

"Give me a hundred bucks and I'll get it."

This is where the real Chicago people came for every imaginable favor. This was, quite simply, where shit got done.

Throw in a father who had no time or inclination to parent, a mom who worked full-time and ran the house—this was Stan, Jr.'s reality. Not ideal, and certainly not the life of privilege his own children would enjoy in later years. In retrospect, Stan often embraced his upbringing. He didn't enjoy it, but he understood it. It defined him and taught him some rough lessons. It was the ultimate school of hard knocks and you better believe that every stinking swabbing of that tavern floor taught him one thing and that was there was something better out there for him that didn't involve mopping up blood, vomit and urine in a tiny shitter on the West Side. What he couldn't know in his young years was that he would wind up in an emergency room that was often loaded with the same blood, urine, and vomit---a more antiseptic environment that the nurses cleaned up.

Stan's mother was not a disinterested party. She knew he was special and brighter than most, if not all, of his peers. He had the 'it' factor and although no one would have called it that in the 1940s and '50s, everyone around him recognized it. He had the leadership bug and was one of those boys born with that elusive alpha male gene that rises to the top of the male DNA pool. People were drawn to him. School was almost a joke. By junior high, he knew he was smarter than most of his teachers. They knew it as well and encouraged him to range outside of the public school curriculum. Make no mistake, this Zydlo kid had 'it' and the West Side was not going to get him.

It was about this time that Stan's mother became desperate. Stan was out of control, fighting, taking on all comers. He was absolutely fearless and would knock you on your ass if you fooled with him. Lots of guys talked a great game, but Stan didn't talk. You wanted some of his narrow, Polish ass, you'd better bring a lunch because he wouldn't quit and he wouldn't ask for mercy.

These events took place on the street, in school and anywhere in between. One event that took place in his front yard at 1473 W. Superior changed his life's trajectory in a way that no one could have guessed. He had just graduated from Motley Grammar School, a few blocks from his home, when the usual end of school year beefs were sorted out by the up and coming neighborhood gangsters. Stan had been in a beef with a local Mexican kid and, as he described it, he had "whooped his ass pretty good."

This was in the late 1940s. People were not getting shot over these minor flare-ups in those years. Nevertheless, this young man wanted a rematch.

He and a few dozen of his closest pals walked over to the Zydlo estate and rang the bell, demanding another shot. Zydlo, who was just sitting down to eat dinner with his Mom and his sister, Geri, shot through the front door and the fight was on. Once again Stan was "wailing the shit out of this guy" and the Mexican kid pulled out a knife and stabbed him in the leg.

Stan's Mom, sitting ringside, was unhappy. It became crystal clear to her that this was the hinge pin event that changed everything. She had thought about this for some time and now she knew what she had to do.

This was the defining moment in Stan's young life, and no one had any idea what a chain reaction this event would cause. Stan had no idea and the neighborhood lightweight champion was about to get a whole new reality. Certainly, the long-forgotten Mexican kid who tried to castrate Zydlo has no idea that he was primarily, indirectly, responsible for saving millions of lives.

Not before, or since, has a front yard fight been the reason for one of the most significant changes in modern medicine. Stan's mother had seen enough. In pre-internet days, one did not just get online and solve a problem. Be that as it may, Mrs. Zydlo was on a mission. She would not watch the next fight where Stan might get himself crippled, or worse yet in her mind, kill someone else and wind up in Statesville penitentiary. However, her husband was not about to pull up stakes and move to Winnetka so Stan, Jr. could attend a nicer, more congenial, school.

Unbeknownst to Stan, the local Polish grocery store owner had a son who had similar issues---fighting and running the streets. Stella Zydlo didn't care if it was Black Jack dealer school. She would get Stan out of the West Side and away from the streets. It pained her to send her bright, precocious son out of state and out of their lives because in many respects it was Stan, Jr. who kept the family moving forward in a positive fashion.

Senior had his politics, his bar, and his excessive, out of control drinking. He was really unplugged from the family. Stella Zydlo did all the heavy lifting. Stan and Geri were the benefactors of her love and protection.

Pain, or no pain, Stan was soon on a bus to sunny Mexico, Missouri and the Missouri Military Academy, an all boys' preparatory boarding school located about as far from the rough and tumble west side of Chicago as one could get.

The Missouri Military Academy (MMA) was about 350 miles from metropolitan Chicago. Traveling in 1948, the bus took about twenty hours to reach the MMA, with what seemed to Stan, Jr. to be 120 stops and no expressways of any kind. When Stan arrived, they were expecting him. When he exited the bus, he thought maybe someone had made a huge mistake. Waiting for him was an old man seated on a horse-pulled wagon. Stan was dumbstruck. He had never seen a horse outside of a racetrack and certainly had never ridden in anything pulled by a horse. He began plotting his getaway.

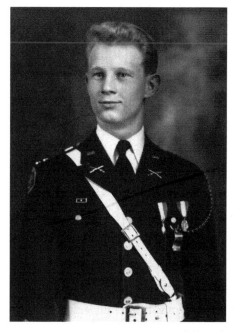

Stan Zydlo circa 1948. Courtesy Zydlo family

He was definitely "not in Kansas anymore." His new surroundings were visually stunning when compared to Chicago. MMA was an excellent academic institution with old-fashioned values. 'Honor, duty, country' was not some corny phrase tossed around at cocktail parties. It was serious business here at MMA and they did not fool around when it came to issues of honor and integrity.

This was 1948 and America was just coming out of a war where, depending on whose stats you believed, the U.S. had lost anywhere from 292,000 to 400,000 men in battles fought across the world. Another 600,000 survived, but returned with various injuries. Over sixteen million Americans served in the war, so there were few families in the entire country that had not been significantly impacted. Patriotism was at an all-time high and the military was revered.

Stan came from an environment where there were really no standards, with the exception of his parish priest at Holy Innocence Church and his mother who attempted to discipline and guide him. In reality, the only standards he was used to were self-imposed ones.

At MMA, there were standards for getting out of bed in the morning. There were rules for everything imaginable and one might think that Zydlo would rebel against seemingly unnecessary rules that governed, for example, how your shoes were to be laced. But the opposite occurred.

Zydlo jumped in with both feet. He loved all of it. The discipline, the uniforms, a chain of command, people who were in your business 24/7--- these were the things that made a huge difference. At this point in his life, this was just what he needed.

His biggest problem was homesickness. A recurring problem for the next eight years was that he was just so damned lonely. He desperately missed his mother and sister. Hell, on occasion, he even missed the old man. But, most of all he missed the neighborhood, his pals, the vibrant city with all its characters, and the ethnic food he grew up on. The first time he saw a bowl of grits, he was amazed that humans actually ate that country shit.

But a transformation was happening. It was something special, almost magical because where he once was teased for getting straight "A's in school, "Hey, genius!" "Hey, super Polack," he was now encouraged. Rather than hiding his report cards and not talking about his grades, he, like everyone at MMA, was smart. It was competitive and it played right into Stan's psyche.

This was what had been missing. Where there was once ridicule and harshness with every comment, there was now encouragement and reward.

He also found out what he didn't realize earlier in life. His peers flocked to him because he had mad leadership skills. His instructors recognized and encouraged it. He had the chops and thrived. He didn't realize it then, but everything he absorbed and experienced at MMA would come in handy throughout his entire life.

It was during this period that a number of unrelated events occurred that would help shape Zydlo's personality and demeanor. Outside of taking a mandatory class of Horsemanship 101, (MMA was still preparing leaders to fight Cavalry style), Stan's Forrest Gump-style existence was starting to amaze him.

His high school years flew by and college approached. By now, Stan was singularly focused on becoming a doctor. At this time in the United States, this was the most prestigious and most difficult goal a young man could have. Medical doctors were revered and respected. They were considered the wise men of society. The American public worshipped their doctors.

Stan had no small goals. He knew he was not returning to Chicago to manage a gin mill and run for an alderman position. He wanted nothing to do with that lifestyle. He was shooting for the top. Nothing less would do.

The question became, "What college gives me the best shot at getting into medical school?"

Neither of his parents had attended college, so they were no help. This was on Stan. Most people reading this today would have no concept of this. Now, parents are far better educated. They understand and recognize how difficult it is to get into a top school. The competition is brutal and kids, from a very young age, are pushed to excel. It is not uncommon for parents to spend hundreds of thousands of dollars on their children's education with the sole goal of getting them into an Ivy League school. In

1952, this was almost unheard of unless a father was an alumnus of Yale, Harvard, or a similar school.

So, Stan began the long and difficult process of figuring this out. Fortunately, he was in the top three or four kids in his class at a highly-rated college prep school. His academic advisor was a pretty hip guy who knew Stan well. He told Stan that if he wanted to go to med school, there was only one place for him. Stan is thinking of Northwestern, or the University of Illinois. "Man, here I come out of the desert, back into the city, the nightlife, man, the girls! Out of purgatory into Heaven."

"Stan, I think you need to apply to Westminster College in Fulton, Missouri."

Zydlo is thinking, "Did I hear this guy right? Did he just say Fulton fucking Missouri? Am I dreaming? Four years in the sticks, no girls and Fulton frigging Missouri?"

His head was spinning. He was not happy. He had just busted his ass for four years so he could get out of this hick town atmosphere and here is this dude telling him, "Hey, four more years of grits for breakfast."

"Where do I sign up?"

Although Zydlo was not happy about the location, there was good news. He knew this was his best option because Westminster was known for its students, as many as seventy-five percent, getting into top flight medical schools. For Zydlo, that was the brass ring and so it was four more years of grits, black-eyed peas and Greyhound bus rides.

He had to work. He needed money for food, so he got a job at nearby William Woods College, a girl's college in Fulton. He worked in the kitchen for three years for the vast sum of a dollar a day ($8.72 a day in today's world). Added onto that was an ROTC scholarship stipend of $27.90 a month ($243.50 a month in today's dollars). Stan was rolling in dough.

Zydlo was a biology and pre-med major at Westminster and working, more or less full-time, at Woods College, so there was not much free time. This would be a recurring theme throughout his life---eighteen to twenty-four hour days would be the norm, but he always felt there were never enough hours in the day. His work ethic continued to be legendary, even among other workaholics. This was just a preview to the next fifty or sixty years.

The academic competition was now serious. All students were motivated and bright. They all had solid backgrounds and many of them were the sons of practicing physicians. Stan was the son of a tavern owner and alderman and that background served him well. He came from a family where you were expected to get things done.

"Hey, get up there and clean the gutters and trim the tree." It didn't matter that you were ten years old and didn't own a ladder. "Figure it out kid. It's not a request. If you don't, I'll be beating your young ass when I get home tonight." Nope, you'd better dummy up as they say in Chicago because if you don't that ass whipping would definitely happen.

Today, we call that child abuse or child neglect. Back then, our parents called it appropriate motivation. It was neither appropriate, nor motivational, but, hey, it worked, most of the time.

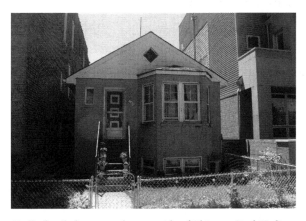

Zydlo family home on the west side of Chicago. Paul Ciolino

Zydlo was not hampered by his chaotic childhood. If anything it served him well. He knew what the wrong side of the tracks looked like and had absolutely no desire to go back there. He was motivated by fear. He did not want to follow in his father's footsteps. First and foremost, he was his own man and thought of himself as a humanist. He was determined. Nothing would stop him. Most assuredly, his background and upbringing were, as far as he was concerned, a non-issue.

As with MMA, Westminster was a great fit for Stan. He thrived and earned straight 'A's in a tough, liberal arts college. He always ranked near the top of his class. He depended on his near photographic memory and always believed he could memorize almost anything he read. In a pre-med curriculum, this was an absolute necessity. Even more critical were the people he met and the friends he accumulated.

When you come from humble beginnings and your family struggles paycheck to paycheck, your whole existence is one of surviving to pay-day. Networking, attending cocktail parties, and hobnobbing with the local big shots is not part of your repertoire. Critical skills that are frequently needed to move onward and upward in life, to open doors, include small talk, being well read and conversant in world affairs. They are often the difference between opportunity and success. Entering MMA, Stan Zydlo's skills included a great left jab and a devastating right hook to the ribs. Simple, but effective only in the street and boxing rings.

Stan didn't realize how quickly he was growing socially. He was well-liked, a class leader who possessed extraordinary honor and commitment qualities. His teachers and deans, who saw it, continually mentored and encouraged him. Life is full of small moments and memories that define us and Stan was no different. Everything that happened to him was a life lesson. He was unaffected by his lack of money and high society contacts.

It was at Westminster one winter evening in 1954 that Stan and recently retired President Harry S. Truman broke bread and bonded. Truman had returned to his hometown of Independence, Missouri. The president of Westminster invited him to the school to give a speech, but no one expected the man who ended World War II by bombing Japan into the Stone Age to show up. But, Harry Truman was not your average politician.

Truman made some of the toughest and most controversial decisions in the history of the U.S. presidency. He fired the very popular General Douglas MacArthur. He integrated the military. He threatened a newspaper reporter who panned his daughter's piano recital. He actually wrote a letter to the critic, told him in writing that he would break his nose, blacken his eyes and perhaps even kick him in the nuts. He did that as a sitting president and without making any apologies.

Truman was poor most of his adult life and as honorable as anyone who ever served as president. His background and upbringing were not a whole lot different than Stan Zydlo's.

While standing in a reception line for President Truman, Stan was talking with him and off to the side was a state senator from Missouri. He had a very young woman with him and it was apparent to Stan and the President that this man wanted to speak to Truman. The President was gracious and clearly interested in Stan and the rest of the students, clearly enjoying the experience.

At some point, the Missouri senator just butted into the conversation. The President looked at him and said, "Goddamit. Son of a bitch, you don't interrupt the President of the United States in that way." He then turned back to Stan and continued to make small talk. Zydlo recalled being in shock and terrified that he had done something wrong.

Later that evening, Truman ate dinner with Stan and apologized for "blowing up" in the reception line. He explained that the senator who interrupted them was not with his wife, but with a girlfriend. Truman was livid because he felt that the senator had tried to use him to show his girlfriend that he and the President were pals. Truman told Stan that there was no chance in hell that he would let that happen.

This event left a lasting impression on Stan as he was shocked that the President preferred eating and talking with him when he could hang out with his admirers. Stan would carry that lesson to his grave. Of course, Truman would always remain his favorite president.

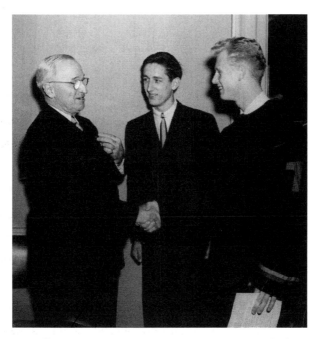

Stan Zydlo and President Harry S. Truman, Courtesy Zydlo family

At Westminster, Stan became very close with Owen Fonkalsrud, a native of Mexico, Missouri and later a prominent psychologist and Army Colonel who lived in Tulsa, Oklahoma. Owen had an uncle named Dr. Nesheon who was a traveling surgeon in Missouri. Owen suggested that if Stan wanted to be a doctor, he might want to meet his uncle and pick his brain.

They met and Dr. Nesheon offered Stan a part-time job helping him on Saturday afternoons while he performed surgeries around the area. Stan jumped at the opportunity and soon was scrubbing in and assisting Dr. Nesheon whenever he could get away. He thought the doctor was a wonderful teacher, very bright and patient.

"He would explain to me exactly when and why we would do something. It was the greatest human anatomy class that one could ever have."

This continued for nearly three years and Zydlo felt he could "absolutely" do this if only he could get into medical school.

The reader might think that Zydlo marched right into medical school and breezed through it. The fact is that Stan came perilously close to not graduating from college at all. During his junior year at Westminster, He applied to medical school at Northwestern and Loyola in Chicago. Loyola interviewed him first and the admissions dean asked Stan after the interview if Loyola was to offer him a slot in medical school, would he accept it? Stan thought about it for about three seconds and said, "Absolutely." The Dean responded, "Welcome to Loyola Medical School. Now all you have to do is graduate and get back to Chicago and start med school." Finally, the long march was nearly over.

Zydlo started his senior year thinking that all he had to do was show up, get decent grades and jump off into medical school. He was pumped and ready, but homesick beyond belief. He wanted to get back to civilization and get on with his life. All he had to do was avoid trouble and take one more long bus ride. He was breezing through senior year when disaster struck.

It wasn't that Stan was having academic issues, it was that the chemistry professor, who was single, decided that to pass his class, Zydlo had to come to his house and stand there while he "felt you up". That would get him a passing grade in a mandatory class. But Zydlo told the professor, "You put one hand on me, I will kick your fat ass all over this campus." By this time, Zydlo had won a Golden Gloves boxing championship in Chicago and was more than happy and capable of backing up his threat.

The professor flunked Zydlo. This set up the proverbial "come to Jesus meeting" with the head of the pre-med program and the university president. Dr. Day, the pre-med director asked Zydlo why he failed to take the chemistry test, why he was throwing his career and graduation down the toilet.

Zydlo replied that he would not take the test and get molested by the chemistry professor if that was what it would take.

The university president questioned Zydlo some more and the next thing Stan knew, without any fanfare or conversation he received a high passing grade and the chemistry professor was gone. Zydlo never took the test and never heard another thing about it. He played the whole thing off as "men being men" and taking care of business. He graduated with honors and went on to medical school.

CHAPTER TWO

"92"

"If you want to make enemies try to change something."
— Woodrow Wilson

It's not his age, it's not his Social Security number, and it's not the four lottery numbers he played on a semi-regular basis. It's not even his Air Force service number. 92---that is his number. You might as well tattoo it on his forehead. He thinks that if he is half-way conscious when he dies, that number---92---may be the last thought he ever has.

On December 1, 1958, a relatively young and soon to be licensed physician named Stanley Zydlo was walking from Loyola Medical School to his home on the west side of Chicago when a Chicago Police motorcycle unit came screaming up next to him and a grizzled, old beat cop said, "Hey, Doc, hop on. We got a really fuckin' bad one." It was probably the most understated comment in the course of modern history.

To provide perspective, 1958 was a pretty interesting time. Elvis Presley was inducted into the Army; Charles DeGaulle and President Eisenhower created NASA, and Saddam Hussein overthrew the Iraqi monarchy and ruled Iraq with an iron fist for more than fifty years. Ted Williams, the last guy to hit .400, was fined $250 for spitting on a fan, which was his second spitting offense, and the U.S. was conducting nuclear tests on a nearly monthly basis. Technology and science were making historic strides, and medicine, in particular, was exploding. Pacemakers were invented, CPR was still two years out, and the brain EEG had been introduced in 1957.

He wasn't a doctor yet, but he had a fairly distinctive medical school uniform that most cops recognized as "doctor clothes." He jumped on the three-wheeler without thinking twice and hung on for dear life, freezing his ass off the entire time as they raced towards what was clearly a sight of Armageddon.

They rolled up to a Roman Catholic grammar school named Our Lady of the Angels, located in a neighborhood known as Humboldt Park. In 1958, it was a working class Italian and Polish neighborhood. Today it is primarily a combat zone for the Latin Kings street gang, the largest Hispanic gang in the country.

Pulling up to the scene was an out of body experience. The school was fully engulfed in a massive fire. Kids jumped out of windows to people standing below. Stan Zydlo saw some of the kids were smoldering. Some bounced off the concrete. It seemed as if every fireman and fire truck in the city was there, as well as police and parents who lived nearby and had smelled the smoke. Some of the parents had hustled home and dragged all manner of ladders to the scene. At one point, there were five thousand people filling the street.

Looking back on that experience, Dr. Zydlo said that the most striking detail---beyond kids being flung out of windows---was that there were well over fifty paddy wagons there to transport the dead and injured, yet few ambulances because they generally moved bodies and little else. The training that the Chicago Fire Department (CFD) and ambulance drivers received was a grand total of eight hours of Red Cross first aid training. At that time, CFD may have owned nine ambulances.

Think about that: a crisis of biblical proportions and not one paramedic or emergency medical technician (EMT) anywhere near this disaster. There was a good reason, though. There was no such thing as a paramedic or EMT at that time because Stan Zydlo had not yet created them. That would change, but it would be another fourteen years to make that change and improvement a working reality.

Trying to describe the scene is like trying to describe what the pits of Hell must look like. This tragedy was very much like the 911 terrorist attack on the Twin Towers in New York City. The body count on September 11. 2001 was much higher, but the Our Lady of the Angels fire involved, almost exclusively, children. Many of their parents were at the scene when they died. The horror of what took place during those three hours was as bad as it gets.

Chicago Firefighter Jack McCone was in command of Squad 6. Upon arriving on scene, several members of Squad 6 quickly unfolded a life net and rushed to catch children jumping from Classroom 211. The moment the children spotted the net, they began to jump so quickly the firemen didn't have time to clear their net before another child landed. Soon they were coming down in multiples making it impossible for the firemen to support the net with all the weight. They were forced to abandon the net to try to catch the children in their arms. The children jumping from Classroom 211 were eighth graders, the largest children in the school, which left firemen like McCone with a double hernia when it was all over.

The fire took the lives of 92 children and three nuns. It would be decades before Stan Zydlo ever got up on a Monday morning and did not for a minute not relive this real, fucking, nightmare. Ninety-two innocent kids with their whole lives ahead of them. How many lives got ruined that day? 184? 1,084? 18,000? No one knows, but you can be fairly certain that anyone who was there and had a front row seat to that hell was never the same again. For Stan, any shred of innocence he may have had left was erased, gone forever. He was twenty-five years old, and would never be the same again.

Zydlo didn't know it yet, but the seed for what would turn out to be a miraculous career had just been planted. Out of one of the biggest, if not the most tragic events that Chicago has ever witnessed, Stanley M. Zydlo, Jr. had just been given the impetus to invent and create the most successful medical branch in the history of modern medicine.

Against all odds, he almost single-handedly would create and train a group of men, and eventually women, who would go on to save millions of lives in the next forty-five years. He would change the face of emergency rooms in every hospital in America. His efforts and his participation would go unnoticed by the public they served. As with every man, woman, and child who was touched by the Our Lady of the Angels fire, this tragedy branded Zydlo's soul. He would be influenced by what he saw that day for the rest of his life. Out of this horrific tragedy the seed was planted that would eventually grow and develop to be the Emergency Medical Service (EMS) system that would save millions of lives across the world.

It is appropriate to consider the part the Our Lady of the Angels fire played in the creation of EMS because publicly, and until this moment, that tragic event has never been associated with anything good or positive. Reading and researching that event makes one realize that the modern world of terror did not begin on September 11. 2001, or only in New York City.

CHAPTER THREE

"All In"

*"Sure, politics isn't bean-bag. 'Tis a man's game, an'women,
childrer, cripples an'prohybitionists'd do well to keep out of iv it."*
– Finley Peter Dunne in an 1895 newspaper column

As you sit in your den or living room here in 2016, you are assured of a number of things. If you turn on a light switch, the light will come on. If you turn on a water faucet, the water will immediately flow. If you dial 911 because you are having a chest pain, an ambulance worth around a million dollars with equipment and at least two highly-trained paramedics will be in your living room within ten minutes, depending upon where you live.

That response time isn't a great standard, but it is certainly better than it was in 1972. The training and equipment however, are the gold standard and we owe that, largely, to Dr. Stan Zydlo.

Prior to, and in 1972, there were no standards. If you were sick, having a heart attack, or badly injured, you had better figure out how to get to a hospital or your doctor's office. If you didn't, the next day you would probably be a dead person. No one got upset or mad, that was simply the way it was.

That isn't entirely true. A number of people thought this was ridiculous. Why in hell could we not treat a heart attack victim in the street? Why couldn't we have trained medical personnel show up at a bad car accident and treat the victims? The reason we could not, as it turned out, was very simple. It was against the law.

The law was clear. Only medical doctors and licensed nurses could treat an injured or sick person. This treatment could only take place in a hospital or doctor's office. If you attempted to do anything beyond that, you could be charged. This was the conundrum. It was a law created by medical professionals that, in Zydlo's opinion, was patently ridiculous. This was where the rubber met the road and everyone seemed paralyzed by it.

Everyone except Stan Zydlo. He grew up in a home where his father was a street savvy Chicago politician who knew how to get things done. Fortunately for the rest of us, Stan, Jr. paid attention during those formative years. He knew what needed to be done and that was a change in the law.

Before he could train one paramedic in CPR, the law had to be changed. No problem, right? We'll mosey on over to the state legislature and tell them to change these silly laws so we can save millions of lives.

In 1972, Zydlo was no longer a "baby doc". He was a force. Thirty-nine and at the top of his game---and he knew it. It was now or never. If he was going to change how business was done, now was the time. He could smell it. Zydlo always thought that life was about "showing up". You have to show up at work, school, your marriage, parenting, whatever. Show up and get involved. Be proactive. Do something,

The fire in '58 that ripped the heart out of anyone it touched, and the funeral home hearses that pulled up to bad traffic accidents waiting for 'customers,' created a tragic comedy of errors that resulted in wasted human life. Thousands who could have, and should have, been saved, goddammit, were left on the side of the road like…fucking road kill.

Call it whatever you want, but for reasons that were crystal clear in Zydlo's mind, Americans had their own Holocaust going on and it was almost as tragic as the one in Hitler's world. Maybe more so because we could actually, with some effort, save hundreds of thousands of lives a year if we could just get enough medical attention to keep people alive until they could be transported to a hospital setting.

Due to medical territorial issues, and just the pure hassle of getting people to move out of their comfort zones, it just wasn't happening. Zydlo and every emergency room doc he knew was seeing the same shit day in and day out. Men and women with serious, yet very treatable injuries were dying like damn dogs because they couldn't get treated in time to save their lives. It was maddening and disgusting.

These thoughts were never far from Stan's mind: "How many have died because nobody was available to help them? How many have become vegetables because there was no one to perform CPR? How many millions have been affected by these injuries? How many parents have buried children because there was no one around to blow a few breaths into an infant's tiny lungs?"

Those were the questions that kept Stan up all night. It is 1972 and Zydlo has reached his limit. As with Julius Caesar crossing the Rubicon in 49 BC, Stan Zydlo was about to cross the medical point of no return. He was going to do the unthinkable. He would take on the entire medical profession and show them how to save lives.

You think the Roman Senate was tough? Try taking on the economic and intellectual juggernaut of the American medical establishment and its professionals. Zydlo knew that a complete paradigm shift at the highest levels of the medical establishment would have to take place.

His employer was supportive to a point. They liked the idea, but as an institution were unwilling to financially back the program. Basically, they were saying to him, "You want to train firemen to be health care professionals? Great. Do it on your own time and do it anywhere but here because we are not getting into a major pissing contest with our doctors." Not exactly a ringing endorsement, but Stan Zydlo would be the linch pin of the entire paramedic machines. His vision, his idea, and most importantly his passion, made it happen.

Historically, medical breakthroughs and advances were discovered in the laboratories and research centers of America. Occasionally a war would necessitate change. In the Korean War, we saw the creation of helicopters being used to lift severely wounded military personnel to Level One trauma centers or field hospitals. In fact, wars have been responsible for incredible advances in medicine. In an article published in 1988, a surgeon, F. William Blaisdell, identified eight medical advances that occurred during the Civil War. These developments involved recordkeeping, management of mass casualties in a timely fashion---the standardization of the ambulance corps being a critical example---design of hospitals, sanitation and hygiene, female nurses, and the vast experience with management, surgery and anesthesia gained by numerous physicians.[1]

As far as Zydlo was concerned, he was in a war right then. All around him people were dropping like flies. In serious accidents, cardiac cases, and drowning incidents, people were more often dead than alive when they arrived in an emergency room. He knew with absolute certainty that thousands, perhaps millions, of lives could be saved if advanced lifesaving techniques were practiced at the scene of these events. Not only was this not happening in 1972, but there was no sense of urgency to begin moving toward a paramedic system.

There had been some attempts in isolated instances. In Ohio, doctors were starting to respond with an ambulance to cardiac events. In Los Angeles and Miami, and other larger cities, there were disjointed efforts to get *something* in place. It was, simply, too overwhelming---too many hurdles, too much politics, too expensive. The list was endless.

Most people would throw up their hands, surrender, stay out of harm's way, and go about their normal lives. Why would a person go through four years of military school, fours of college, four years of medical school, more years of training and internships, a three-year stint in the U.S. Air Force, and then piss off everyone who could make his life miserable and perhaps ruin his career and life? Why would anyone take that chance?

Fortunately for those of us who have been on the receiving end of the Paramedic/EMT lifesaving efforts, Stan Zydlo decided to roll the dice and fight the fight that needed a warrior, though hospitals aren't exactly the place one would look for a warrior. Certainly, there are rare exceptions, but most doctors did not spend the majority of their life killing themselves to throw it all away on a "cause".

Stan could feel it this time. He woke up every day thinking about it. He could not get it done by telling people what needed to be done. He was approaching it incorrectly. This was simple, he thought. Quit talking about it. Let the housewife talk. It's time to act.

The "housewife" was the hyperactive Janet L. "Jan" Schwettman, of Inverness, an upper middle class suburb of Chicago, who began showing up everywhere. Stan thought she was a huge pain in the ass, but people were actually paying attention to her. She was not political or a gadfly. She had no agenda, not married to a doctor or fireman. She was simply a very bright woman who happened to have a friend whose 43-year-old husband had a heart attack and tragically died in their living room in August 1971 with members of the fire department unable to render meaningful assistance.

This was nothing new. People had been dropping dead in their homes since the beginning of time. This time, however, the frustration level boiled over, the proverbial straw that broke the camel's back. The beginning of a perfect storm that resulted in Mrs. Schwettman and Dr. Zydlo coming together.

On January 12, 1972, Jan was at Northwest Community Hospital talking with Dr. Marjorie Smith who introduced her to Dr. Zydlo. They immediately discovered their mutual goal and a partnership of sorts was born.

Both Schwettman and Zydlo campaigned and appeared in front of local village boards attempting to secure funding for the program. On occasion, they got commitments fairly quickly, but there was resistance in some quarters.

Schwettman was everywhere, in constant motion, talking to anyone who had anything to do with heart attacks, first aid, or emergency rooms. She met with Captain Jack Benson in Arlington Heights, who was trying to start an advanced life support system. She found that many of the firemen were as frustrated with the system as she was.

Primarily financed by her own money, Schwettman crisscrossed the country with some small contributions that trickled in from people aware of her missionary zeal to get a program established. She talked to experts who had started, or were attempting to start, similar programs. She spoke with Dr. Eugene Nagel and Dr. James Warren at a conference in Pittsburgh, Pennsylvania, both of whom had programs, but not as all-inclusive as Dr. Zydlo planned. She gathered steam and friends in high places, quickly becoming the civilian expert on these matters.

Dr. Zydlo watched with interest, thinking Schwettman might finally push them over the edge. He was in the initial stages of creating a training program that would become the model for EMTs and paramedics. This group would not be the first in the United States, but when they finished they would be the best trained and the future model for all of those who followed. Dr. Zydlo's model was solely based on what *he* thought would work and what *he* thought was needed.

There were no committees, no advisors, no protocol written or suggested. There were zero experts to consult. No one from the hospital offered suggestions. Hell, the hospital administration appeared to be for the program, but they actively hedged their bets, offered little help and absolutely no guidance. They initially refused to let Dr. Zydlo conduct training at the hospital or even copy training materials there. They gave public lip service, but privately stood back and watched to see which way the wind would blow. In a final insult, they suggested that Zydlo should take a leave of absence while he trained the firemen, but didn't suggest how he should feed his family while conducting the training.

Together with Jan Schwettman and a few Chicago suburban fire chiefs, Zydlo started a full court press to establish some sort of emergency medical mobile service to reach severely ill or injured persons and save their lives. This service was meant to aid them while they were transported to a "real medical facility" to receive first class medical treatment.

Columbus, Ohio; Seattle, Washington; and a few California cities were attempting to put together some sort of mobile lifesaving apparatus, but it is without question that Dr. Zydlo, Schwettman and those first brave firefighters were successful in putting together the first multi-jurisdictional medical centers and emergency medical technicians-paramedics who could perform advanced medical techniques in the streets. They were not doctors or nurses.

They did this on guts, not knowing the outcome, challenges or obstacles that would be thrown in their path. They were exactly what has made this country the finest example of what is good and honorable in this world. Certainly no one realized what this paramedic thing would grow into.

Their efforts back in 1972 would eventually evolve into a medical practice that would equal the discovery of Penicillin or the measles vaccine.

CHAPTER FOUR

Genesis

"Genius inspires resentment. A sad fact of life."
– Eoin Colfer

No one, literally no one, liked this paramedic talk. Who's going to pay for it? Who's going to do the training? Who's going to supply the training? Who's going to determine what the training standards are? Who will license and administer the program? Who will be responsible for any liability issues? Who will decide what the standard of care is? Endlessly the list went on.

Who indeed? For a moment consider the magnitude of putting together a system that is geared towards saving lives in any condition imaginable. In your home, in the factory, on the street, at the mall, on a ballfield or in a park. During thunderstorms, in the heat, during a blizzard, 24/7 no break no relief. A call for help comes in and the apparatus springs to life. Simple enough today in 2016. In 1972, impossible. There was no system. There were no paramedics. Very few people had even thought about how you would do all this.

But Stan Zydlo had thought about it and thought about it, and considered every angle from which to attack the problem. He knew that he alone would be taking the heat for anything that went wrong. He knew that the training of the paramedics had to be perfect. In the end the trueness of the program, the excellence had to come from its inventor. Zydlo knew that excellence came from the amount of heart you put into anything you did. It did not matter if it was boxing or medicine. It had to be true and it had to be pure. In the end, that trueness could only come from within. The paramedics had to have the heart of Zydlo in the street. He thought that if he could install this in his paramedics the whole thing would eventually fall into place.

The mere idea of putting what is now known as Emergency Medical Services (EMS) together was overwhelming. All of the aforementioned were very valid points and the simple and glaring fact was implementing and getting the EMS up and running was not going to happen without super human efforts, genius, and money. A lot of money, and a few geniuses, would get it up and running. Sustaining and running the program would require nothing short of a miracle.

Start with the 911 system that we have today. It works and it is brilliantly effective. The number of lives it has saved is in the millions. Only problem is, the system that we have today really didn't exist in 1972. So, not only was there no EMS system there was no 911 to get them there if they did exist.

If you are starting to figure out what Stan Zydlo had to overcome to get what he envisioned up and running, you have an idea how this project destroyed Zydlo's health and gave him his first heart attack at age forty-one, about six years after the Northwest Suburban EMS was up and running. In fact, had Stan not recruited the local fire departments to help and eventually supply almost all of the personnel, the EMS system would have died on the table. In addition to the fire departments, there were two private ambulance companies and one police department. The original and charter towns/entities were:

1. Arlington Heights Fire Department
2. Buffalo Grove Fire Department
3. Hoffman Estates Fire Department
4. Mount Prospect Fire Department
5. Morton Grove Fire Department
6. Palatine Fire Department
7. Rolling Meadows Fire Department
8. Schaumburg Fire Department
9. Lake Zurich Police Department
10. Delta Ambulance Service
11. Arlington Ambulance

With the exception of the private ambulance companies who sent limited personnel, these northwest suburbs of Chicago at the time were quite small and had limited resources and money. They are certainly not the powerhouse towns that they are today.

In retrospect there are some very good reasons that the EMS system was not developed in a major city. Costs, politics, know how, a hundred different reasons why it couldn't be done. The original participating towns, villages, cities listed here were just affluent enough to swing the initial costs. They all had a fairly substantial middle to upper middle class population that was well educated. The fire departments and specifically the chiefs could see the handwriting on the wall that there was not a whole lot of fires being fought. It was time to diversify and what better way then to implement a whole new breed of firemen?

The biggest hurdle perhaps would be the public trust. Will they buy it? Will they support it? The other issue facing Zydlo was a legal one. It was a simple legal issue, which was a huge problem because what Dr. Zydlo was proposing was literally *illegal*. In the state of Illinois, it was against the law for anyone beside doctors and nurses to perform any medical services outside of a medical facility or doctor's office.

There were other agencies, and some medical doctors, who were experimenting with a full service paramedic service. Certainly, Los Angeles was as close as anyone to instituting a full paramedic service and that was driven by a fictional television show called *Emergency*, which aired in 1972. The show was so popular that the politicians in Los Angeles started clamoring for an actual paramedic service. Dr. Zydlo sent two of his paramedics, Dale Collier, from Palatine and Berny Goss, from Elk Grove Village, to advise them on some of the shows.

The credit for who instituted the first full service emergency management system has often been totally inaccurate. Research today discloses very inaccurate data. For example, on the website "The virtual EMS museum" (http://www.emsmuseum.org/virtual-museum/history), their website states that Dr. David Boyd did the following:

"By 1974, Dr. Boyd's trauma system had become fully operational. Based on that success, he was appointed by the President of the United States to serve as Chief of the Department of Health, Education and Welfare (HEW) Emergency Medical Services (EMS) Division. He applied the success from Illinois with a vision of building "wall-to-wall" EMS systems throughout the country. He travelled extensively and personally met with local EMS leaders. His program built upon the successes of the previous Robert Wood Johnson Foundation grants for regional communications systems."

The above statement is not factually true and it is very misleading with regard to who started and implemented the paramedic system that we enjoy today. Dr. Stanley M. Zydlo, Jr., MD was the founder and creator of the first fully operational EMS system and trained paramedic system in the United States.

Zydlo's system was on line and operating by December 1, 1972. Dr. Boyd was not within fifty miles of this operation. Although Boyd very well may have done what is written above he was late to the game. By 1974, Zydlo's program had been up and running for over a year. The State of Illinois initially had zero jurisdiction over Zydlo's EMS system.

It was not until August 1973 that the state started testing and licensing paramedics. The first state paramedic test occurred at Northwest Community Hospital on August 15, 1973. Prior to that time, Dr. Zydlo was the sole authority and tester of any paramedic candidates. He developed and instituted the first protocol and training methods. All other programs were a reflection of Zydlo's standards and requirements. Dr. Boyd was a surgeon and was involved, but not as the creator and father of the system. Dr. Boyd worked for the State of Illinois, Department of Public Health and later became a huge contributor but he *was not* by any means the founding father of the program.

Not only was Boyd not the founder of this system, but he actually sent down an underling to tell Zydlo that the paramedics should not be giving IVs and should not be shocking patients and on and on, and so forth. Zydlo responded by telling him, "Well, should we let them die then?" That was the end of directives from Boyd to Zydlo.

Early newspaper articles clearly state and indicate that Zydlo was the father of the EMS system.

<u>**The Salt Lake City Times**</u>, 04/02/72, "

<u>**The Herald/Buffalo Grove, 12/04/72**</u>, Paramedic Idea pays off-Woman's life Saved" Dr. Zydlo who is in charge of training the paramedics"

The Daily Herald, 11/30/73, "Area paramedics; the real life savers". "Northwest suburban network first to include more than one town in a single system".

The Herald/Wheeling, 11/30/73, "Suburban paramedics bring em back alive" "Dr. Zydlo the tireless director of the program"

Chicago Tribune, 04/04/74, "Paramedics have proven worth in Northwest suburbs, Dr. Zydlo started the training program for paramedics".

Chicago Sun-Times, 01/93, "20 Yrs Ago, Doctor Came to Paramedics' Aid"

Daily Herald Newspaper, 10/08/94, "Doctor Wins National Award for paramedic work".

Daily Herald Newspaper 11/22/97, "Father of paramedic system honored".

Wikipedia offers how they think the first paramedic program was developed:

"New York City's Saint Vincent's Hospital developed the United States' first Mobile Coronary Care Unit (MCCU) under the medical direction of William Grace, MD, and based on Frank Pantridge's MCCU project in Belfast, Northern Ireland.[when?] In 1967, Eugene Nagle, MD and Jim Hirschmann, MD helped pioneer the United States' first EKG telemetry transmission to a hospital and then in 1968, a functional paramedic program in conjunction with the City of Miami Fire Department. In 1969, the City of Columbus Fire Services joined together with the Ohio State University Medical Center to develop the "HEARTMOBILE" paramedic program under the medical direction of James Warren, MD and Richard

Lewis, MD. In 1969, the Haywood County (NC) Volunteer Rescue Squad developed a paramedic program under the medical direction of Ralph Fleicher, MD. In 1969, the initial Los Angeles paramedic training program was instituted in conjunction with Harbor General Hospital under the medical direction of Michael Criley, MD and James Lewis, MD. In 1969, the Seattle "Medic 1" paramedic program was developed in conjunction with the <u>Harborview Medical Center</u> under the medical direction of Leonard, Cobb. The Marietta (GA) initial paramedic project was instituted in the Fall of 1970 in conjunction with Kennestone Hospital and Metro Ambulance Service, Inc. under the medical direction of Luther Fortson, MD. The Los Angeles County and City established paramedic programs following the passage of The Wedsworth-Townsend Act in 1970. Other cities and states passed their own paramedic bills, leading to the formation of services across the US. Many other countries also followed suit, and paramedic units formed around the world."

Much of this is factual, but there is a glaring omission and that is that Zydlo and the Northwest EMS system went on line on Dec 1, 1972. The significant differences between Zydlo's EMS and all of the others was the total package of training that he put his paramedics through.

The actual functions that the paramedics performed in the field were quickly becoming epic. Zydlo's paramedics were far and away the best trained and had far more autonomy and responsibility then any other paramedics or EMT's of that time period. The communications that they employed, and multi-jurisdictional nature of his program that had multiple separate cities and towns working under one umbrella, initially stood alone. Others were kicking the tires and test driving, but nobody had taken it to Zydlo's level.

These features are what separated Zydlo's program from all others and the fact is no program was even close to what Zydlo had cooking in the Northwest suburbs of Chicago in 1972. There certainly weren't any paramedic programs that reached the medical level of Zydlo's paramedics.

It is true that California passed the first law (The Wedsworth-Townsend Act of 1970) authorizing paramedics to perform pre-hospital care but Dr. Zydlo's program was in fact the first fully operational program. Zydlo's program was so magnificently successful that he quickly became the most sought after speaker in the country. Everyone, and I mean every town and city in America, wanted in on this whole ambulance/paramedic thing.

Near the end of the first year in operation, (1973) Zydlo and the paramedics had racked up an incredible record of service and excellence. The ten towns in the system went from primarily transporting victims and giving them oxygen, (regardless of what their ailment was) to treating and saving the lives of victims. At the end of that first year, they had treated and transported 6850 patients.

The breakdown was:

Auto Accident	1795
Other Injury	1993
Cardiac	841
Medical Emergency	1777
Overdose	404
Obstetric	40

The critics and naysayers were quickly becoming a distant memory. The media loved the program and the paramedics were the new darlings of the first responder community. Stan Zydlo, though, was not having much fun. Between being on call non-stop 24/7 he was still at war with his medical colleagues. They, well, they were not happy. This Zydlo guy was a pain in the ass. He made all of them look like shit. We look like clowns and we were dead wrong.

Someone had to pay and Zydlo was the whipping boy.

Zydlo may have been a rock star in the growing EMS community, but in his world of medicine he was being frozen out socially and professionally. Outside of the emergency room and the ambulances, there was no love for the brilliant Dr. Zydlo and as far as he was concerned he did not have one extra minute in his life to deal with whom or who did not receive credit. It was now about the paramedics and it was just that simple.

He was so busy working and sharing the Gospel of Zydlo that he had absolutely zero patience for anything that did not contribute to or help his paramedic program. This would prove to be a mistake when looking at the program and his work from a historical perspective. Now forty-four plus some odd years later we are attempting to set that record straight. Had Zydlo published a couple of articles in medical journals this point might be mute.

His critics were not going to do it for him and at the end of the day he always felt that he was in the life saving business not the "How will history view me in a hundred years?" business. That is not what drove him and I hope, with time, he will be appropriately remembered by those outside of the EMS community.

Zydlo was the heart and soul of the paramedic program, but Jan Schwettman was the driving raging force behind the legislation that allowed a paramedic system to become a reality. Schwettman and Zydlo were the perfect storm that came together and simply made it all happen. Zydlo was tired of talk and he wanted action. Schwettman became the lobbyist, the unelected politician who dogged the Illinois legislature into submission.

Jan Schwettman was a housewife and Mom. She lived in Inverness, an upper middle class suburb of Chicago and she was not political or a gadfly of any type. She had no agenda. She was not married to a doctor or fireman. She was simply a very bright woman who happened to have a friend whose 43-year old husband had a heart attack and tragically died in their living room in August of 1971, with members of the fire department unable to render any meaningful assistance.

This was nothing new as people had been dropping dead in their homes since the beginning of time. This time, however, the frustration level boiled over. It was the proverbial straw that broke the camel's back. It was the first part of the perfect storm that resulted in Mrs. Schwettman and Dr. Zydlo coming together.

In the following weeks and months, Jan Schwettman was everywhere. She was in constant motion and talking to anyone who even remotely had anything to do with heart attacks, first aid, emergency rooms, etc.

Both Schwettman and Zydlo campaigned and appeared in front of local village boards attempting to secure funding for the program. On occasion, they got commitments fairly quickly, but there was still resistance in some quarters.

Everything started to come together. Dr. Zydlo was in the initial stages of putting together a training program that would become the model for EMTs and paramedics. This group would not be the first EMTs and paramedics in the United States, but when they finished they would be perhaps the best trained and the future model for all of their successors. Dr. Zydlo's model was solely based on what *he* thought would work and what *he* thought was needed.

There were no committees, no advisors, and no protocol written or suggested. There were zero experts to consult. No one from the hospital offered suggestions. Hell, the hospital appeared to be for this, but they were actively hedging their bets and offering very little help and absolutely no guidance. They initially refused to let Zydlo conduct training at the hospital. They wouldn't even let Zydlo copy training materials there. No, the hospital was publicly giving lip service, but privately they were standing back watching to see which way the wind would blow. In a final insult, they suggested to Dr. Zydlo that he perhaps should take a leave of absence while he was training the firemen. They didn't suggest how he should feed his family while he was conducting this training.

In many ways the program was constantly on life support those first few years and once it was up and running it was still operating in a crisis mode while everyone except Zydlo and the paramedics were waiting to see how long it would take for a paramedic to kill someone. The politics of this thing were at times overwhelming. Dr. Zydlo mostly shielded the paramedics. Politically, he did the heavy lifting and kept the wolves at bay.

The paramedics in some departments weren't exactly winning friends and influencing people as easily as you might expect. In Rolling Meadows, there was some serious acrimony early on because of Chief Fogarty's initial resistance. That changed after his paramedics saved his life, but there was still a strong division.

In one particular exchange, one of the firefighters was bitching about hoses and water and how much tougher they had it physically over the paramedics. An unidentified paramedic quipped, "We run more fluid through IV tubes then you guys run water through fire hoses in a year".

In Morton Grove, IL the Chief flat out hated the program. Nevertheless, the paramedics were doing God's work out there and gathered fans quicker then Elvis did in Tupelo on a good weekend. In Elk Grove Village, the paramedics were running ten trips to every one that the fire department ran for fires or fire alarms. Considering that Elk Grove had the largest industrial park in the United States, that is quite a fact. It quickly became apparent to anyone with a calculator that the paramedic mission was becoming *the* mission in the fire departments.

This multi town, multi-jurisdictional formation was huge. This is what really separated Zydlo's plan from everyone else. In addition, Zydlo's paramedics would be given more training and have far more responsibility than had anyone to date. There were numerous attempts at putting something similar together, but no one, to date, had all the components of Dr. Zydlo's plan. Zydlo's model would far and away exceed anything that had been attempted so far. It would, in fact, become the model for every EMS program in the country. This was the big-ticket item that would change the face of modern medicine.

CHAPTER FIVE

The Chiefs

"True Heroism is unremarkably sober, very undramatic.
It is not the urge to surpass all others at whatever cost,
but the urge to serve others at whatever cost."
– Arthur Ashe

These guys were not to be trifled with. This was definitely a mixed bag of nuts. These fire chiefs were like a big old burlap sack full of rattlesnakes. You stick your hand in there and you would definitely get bit. But, they were, to a man, old school smoke eaters. Oxygen tank? Little girls wear oxygen tanks. Firemen suck that shit in and spit it out. No, these guys were men in every sense of the word. They came from a time and era where your word was your bond, and your handshake was a solemn oath.

They were not yet quite in the modern age with the high tech equipment that is around today. They fooled around with some pretty antique equipment. The mayors and city managers thought of their paid professional firefighters as a necessary evil. Their benefits and their pensions were a gigantic pain in the ass. The chiefs? They were all skilled street fighters. They knew how to get shit done. They had sharp elbows and were not afraid to throw them.

This Dr. Zydlo guy---they did not know. They knew very little about him. He was a little too confident, a little too cocky. Let's see if we have this right. Zydlo plans to teach our guys (who have zero medical experience) how to save lives. He will teach them how to shove a big plastic tube down people's throats, and stick needles in their veins and arteries. He will teach them how to save heart attack victims, drowning victims, traffic accident victims with arms and legs torn off, and every other conceivable injury or emergency, and he's going to do it in less than six months?

Some of the chiefs were not thrilled with these activities. Their first thought was "What happens when one of my firemen accidentally sticks that plastic tube in the wrong spot and kills someone? Where is this Zydlo dude going to be then? It's all well and good to do these things in an emergency room with trained doctors and nurses under bright lights, with the latest equipment, but what happens when you are in a public housing unit, with no electricity, no help, and surrounded by a hostile gang, cockroaches, and drunk, high or psycho family members? Zydlo won't be holding your hand and pulling armed security to cover your back. Nope, he's going to be sitting in his nice little warm emergency room, surrounded by hot nurses, and drinking cocoa."

Larry Pairitz had been the chief of the Mount Prospect Fire Department since 1970. Like most everyone in that time period, he started as a volunteer fireman and then became a full-time paid fireman in 1961. He was one of the younger chiefs, smart and progressive. He saw the writing on the wall and read the tea leaves. All clues leaned toward a far different fire department than when he came on the job. The community was growing by leaps and bounds. There were major tollways and roads running through town. The department was busy responding to more and more accidents that required substantial first aid of some type. Soon, eight hours of Red Cross First Aid training would not be enough.

In late 1971 or early '72, Chief Pairitz sent two firemen, Ken Koeppen and Lowell Fell, to Loyola Medical Center for an Emergency Medical Technician (EMT) course. Koeppen and Gibson came back and were very enthusiastic about the training and the potential for helping people. That was all Chief Pairitz needed to hear. He was off and running. In his mind, there was no turning back.

Pairitz called people in the community to inquire as to who could teach a local EMT course. Very early on, he spoke with a woman who was somewhat of a community activist. Her name was Mitzie Vavra. Mitzie was a volunteer at Northwest Community Hospital. She told Pairitz that he should probably speak to a Doctor Stan Zydlo. She warned him that Zydlo liked to use pretty colorful language. Pairitz assured her that the firemen could tolerate the language.

Pairitz was a younger chief, at the start of his chief career. Most of the older chiefs in the area were not interested in gearing up for the next big change. They were old smoke eaters who did not see the need for a whole "new branch" in the fire service. This was a war they were not very interested in fighting. Nevertheless. many of the politicians were and they basically funded and ordered the reluctant chiefs into the EMT/Paramedic program. But, in the beginning it was primarily Pairitz who had the vision.

Today, Pairitz poo-pahs his role. Maybe it's the Midwest upbringing, or his conservative middle class values. The men who started this program all seem to be programmed along the same lines. Dr. Zydlo was perhaps a little bit too much Hollywood. He did seem to like the media and the lime-light a little bit too much for the taste of some of the chiefs. But, Zydlo and Pairitz knew the program had to be sold and the public had to have an idea what this whole "paramedic thing" was about.

As soon as Chief Pairitz got together with Dr. Zydlo the plan started to change. Zydlo was very willing to teach a local EMT class for just the Mt.

Prospect Fire Department, but he had already started to plan a much larger multi-department system involving multiple agencies and a much more advanced model of first responders called paramedics. Along with Jan Schwettman, Dr. Zydlo was already recruiting and politicking this thing. Pairitz readily agreed to the upgraded version of what he proposed and supplied the space for the initial classes.

Zydlo tended to move at warp speed in everything he did. Getting this program up and running required an even bigger sense of urgency. Part of his strategy was to shock and awe everyone. He did not want the bureaucrats to have time to think. He did not want to hear from the naysayers, the folks who were incapable of making decisions quickly. He especially did not want the hospital attorneys or city legal counsel to think about potential liability. If the lawyers got involved in the decision process, this whole program would die before the first official call for help. The minute some corporate committee became involved was when everything would grind to a halt.

With the chiefs firmly in camp, Zydlo added a whole bunch more arrows to his quiver. The chiefs were pretty clueless what this was going to mean long term. Certainly no one even began to guess what a juggernaut this would turn into. Did anyone even suspect that one day the fire department paramedics would be doing five and a half million chest pain runs every year? Add other trauma and accidents and you are talking about a commitment that no one could foresee.

Consider that this whole paramedic thing was untested, unproven and in the mind of the medical community, heresy. With the exception of a few isolated places scattered around the country, no one was considering something of this magnitude. Dr. Zydlo worked the chiefs hard. He was a whirlwind and just simply wore them down. He convinced them that this was the way to go and their firemen were the guys who could do it.

If you were walking down the street and ran into **Ted Loesch**, you would not be particularly impressed. He doesn't stand out. He is a typical looking, older, white guy. Not too tall, average build, mustache, and quick to smile. He almost looks like a tough guy version of Floyd the Barber from the Andy Griffin TV show. Yet, something quickly separates him from other people---if you are having a heart attack in your living room, Ted Loesch is exactly the guy you want to show up. Loesch had a switch and when it got hit he jumped right into the middle of a tragedy. You'd be damned impressed, then.

Ted was in the first class of paramedics that Zydlo trained. One year later, he became chief of the Rolling Meadows, Illinois Fire Department. Five years prior, he had been a barber in Rolling Meadows. He will tell you one thing today that he never forgot. He knew a lot more about hairstyles than performing CPR and saving lives. But, Ted Loesch had that special something, that quality that since the beginning of time every child yearned and searched for in their father's character. He had hero quality. The ability to jump into the middle of any tragedy and make it better. He was, and still is, at a fairly advanced age, a stone cold, real deal heroic figure that if required could still perform to standard. To this day, Ted Loesch is still a stud.

Retired from the fire service since 2000, he still has the "Right Stuff". You can feel his vibe, his quiet confidence, and see the whip smart intelligence in his eyes. He is still a physical specimen, great shape, no fat on him, and an iron grip. He is the quintessential American success story. Married to Marge for over fifty years, they raised a platoon of public servants. Two of their sons were Marines and firemen. One of their grandsons is an active duty Marine stationed at Twenty-Nine Palms and headed to Okinawa.

Ted and Marge have lived in the same simple, but beautiful, small, single-story ranch for over fifty years. They attend Mass without fail every

Sunday. They live two blocks from the firehouse. Behind their house, attached to the garage, is a beautiful room that displays his fishing trophies and a big, old-fashioned barber chair. Ted still cuts hair.

When Loesch, the younger, did not see a future for himself in Highland Park, he left the country and moved to Rolling Meadows, a town that could not be further culturally from Highland Park than New York City is from Tupelo, Mississippi.

As the popular town barber, Ted's barbershop was gossip central and a popular destination for the largely volunteer firemen in town. Ted made a great living. He liked his job and the human interaction. Ted liked the firemen whose hair he cut, liked the idea of hanging out with them, so on March 1, 1962, he started his career with the Rolling Meadows Fire Department as a volunteer fireman. In 1968, he became a full-time paid fire fighter.

The starting pay was eight thousand dollars a year. You were paid once a month. Loesch took a huge pay cut. This was a recurring theme with many of these men and was why so many of them had second and third jobs. This firefighting business was fun, adventurous, and exciting at times, but man it paid shit.

If you were badly injured or experiencing a cardiac event of any consequence, you'd better pray that you got to a hospital and found a really good emergency doctor on duty because the fire department personnel were primarily around to transport you. That's it. No First Aid, no IV's, nothing---except, perhaps oxygen.

Ted Loesch is a charter member of the first paramedic course. He went from fireman/paramedic to Fire Chief/Paramedic in a little under a year. Part of this was due to the fact Fire Chief Tom Fogarty (Ted's boss) was lying in bed on August 16, 1973, (8 1/2 months after the paramedics hit the street) when Mrs. Fogarty called the fire station and told Ted that she thought her husband was having a heart attack. Years before Ted had attended a CPR class, (on his own time and expense) and Fogarty had flat out ordered Loesch to not "perform CPR under any circumstances" because he (Fogarty) did not want Loesch to break any ribs on any of the town residents. Never mind that they would die without CPR, the potential rib fracturing was a deal breaker for Fogarty.

Because of Zydlo and Loesch, the ironies of irony occurred when Fogarty went down with a massive heart attack and Loesch, Cooney, Bills, and Dr. Zydlo saved his life, less than a year into the program.

When Loesch and his partners, Bob Cooney and Harold Bills, arrived at the Chief's house he was in full cardiac arrest. He was not breathing, his lips were blue and for all practical purposes he was dead as a mackerel. Loesch and Cooney started CPR. They got the ER on the radio and followed Zydlo's protocol. They transmitted data and pulled out all the stops to save Fogarty.

Fogarty was responding and not saying shit about the CPR compressions. The problem was with the hospital. The radio communications were sketchy at best. Loesch, Cooney, and Bills worked frantically. The ER Doc insisted that they transport Fogarty "immediately". Loesch refused. The paramedics wanted to stabilize him further. Loesch had one of the guys call Dr. Zydlo to have him meet them at the hospital. Zydlo told them to keep doing what they were doing and he would meet them at Northwest Community and take over.

Fogarty survived and eventually retired. He and Loesch were never close, primarily due to Fogarty's stubborn opposition to the paramedic program. Fogarty could not see beyond the potential liability. He wanted nothing to do with this "paramedic nonsense". Zydlo by-passed him and went straight to the city council and mayor. They got it.

Fogarty was 51 at the time of his heart attack. His father had died at a very young age of a heart attack. After shocking Fogarty three times, they finally got him going again. Eventually three other firemen, Donald Gustafson, Roger Hugg, and Ray Weiner, showed up to assist. After Loesch and the other paramedics saved him, Fogarty suddenly became a fan. He also started to rewrite history when interviewed about his close call. Suddenly, he was always "all for it".

For Ted Loesch, the Fogarty episode was one of the most memorable early saves. Throughout the next thirty years, there would be hundreds more. Chief Loesch was a star as a paramedic. He was a charter member of the first paramedic class and he knew exactly how valuable and lifesaving the program had become. Man, he lived to pump the life back into a critically injured or sick person. It was the height of being a professional and as time and experience began to pile up, Loesch became a force.

He spread the word throughout the community. He lectured at PTA, women's groups, etc. Everybody was apprehensive. "You mean you guys are not doctors?" "You're going to see my underwear?" They were all suspicious and not at all appreciative of the skill set the firemen/paramedics now possessed. This was part of the early struggle for acceptance. The media coverage was turning around, word was getting out, and attitudes were slowly changing.

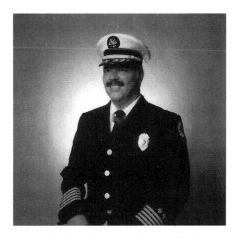

Rolling Meadows IL Fire Chief and inaugural paramedic class member Ted Loesch
Courtesy Ted Loesch

Loesch realized very early on that the fire service of old was in trouble. Building codes, sprinkler systems, and flame retardant materials were making house fires obsolete. There were still fires, there always would be, but they were a fraction of what they were in the old days. The paramedic service quickly became the overwhelming value to the community---a 'must have' service in every town, city, and burg. It was a transitional time in the fire departments and chiefs like Loesch recognized this early on. Loesch's intuition would prove to be spot on.

Professionally, Ted's life was great. Rolling Meadows and the fire department were doubling in size. Personally, it was great, as well, until one evening in March 1974 when Marge was bathing their seven-year-old son, Tommy, and saw he was covered in bruises. Ted and Marge questioned Tommy who denied falling or doing anything that would cause all the bruising. They took him to Northwest Community and discovered he had acute childhood leukemia. Like any parents would be, Ted and Marge were dumbstruck.

The prognosis was acutely critical. Tommy was so sick he was not expected to live more than a few days. As many first responders throughout the years have discovered, you are not immune to these tragedies. Still that does not make it any easier to deal with.

Dr. Zydlo was in the emergency room sewing up an older lady's foot. She was face down on a gurney while he cleaned and stitched a nasty cut. A nurse assisted him. The patient carped about the pain, the stitches, the room temperature, and anything else she could think to bitch about.

When Ted found Stan in the ER, he walked into a curtained off area and without any ceremony told him about Tommy. The older lady quickly shut up. She listened to this tragedy play out above her cut up foot and apparently decided that perhaps her problems were not so bad. Zydlo continued to work on her foot while he discussed options with Ted. He never raised his voice, never hesitated.

He located and made arrangements with a medical school friend, a highly regarded oncologist, to recommend a more qualified medical facility. In spite of how devastated Ted was, he could not help but notice that Dr. Zydlo never took his eyes off what he was doing, but thought through the problem while sewing up the lady and telling his nurse to contact Dr. Joe Simone. They got Tommy into the University of Illinois hospital where he was able to survive another several months before the cancer tragically took him.

Ted and Marge never forgot how Stan Zydlo responded to their family tragedy. Stan was the head of the paramedic tribe and as the chief there was nothing he would not do for a member. This was not an unusual act of kindness on his part, this is who he was---and his paramedics were just like him. This was the type of relationships the paramedic service was built upon.

Unlike most familial tragedies that occur privately among blood relations, the relationship between Zydlo and the paramedics often ran hotter and deeper. They were built and bonded over tragedy and often in the ecstasy of pulling people back from the brink of death. They jointly participated in these catastrophic accidents and injuries, resurrecting dead people in a team effort. This, combined with the political fight that was always humming away in the background of what they were doing, built an incredible bond between the men that became the overriding factor in everything they did.

The paramedics quickly figured out that Dr. Zydlo would do anything for them. He would cut their heart out if they screwed up, but he would still love them and fight for them.

Stan realized that he was extremely tough on his paramedics, but he saw what they were accomplishing. He also knew what they were sacrificing. The stress, the hours, the low pay, the often ungrateful public and bosses. The bad list was never ending. Stan would not hesitate when they needed him. This was in his DNA. He could not change if he wanted to.

In the full circle that we often witness in life, Ted Loesch would eventually help Stan Zydlo bury three of his own children. For over forty years they fought like St. Francis of Assisi to save lives. They did it in every conceivable way. In the end, they had to watch four of their own children die. It was in the end however, that they still found their beginning.

The Arlington Heights Fire Department (AHFD) was, and still is, the largest department in the Northwest Illinois EMS system. Arlington Heights is an upper middle class community of over seventy-five thousand, northwest of Chicago and about three miles from O'Hare International Airport. It is, by population, the largest suburb of Chicago. Of the original inaugural paramedic class taught by Dr. Zydlo, Mt. Prospect Fire Department graduated the most, with seventeen.

Today, AHFD has 110 employees, with four fire stations. Its chief is **Ken Koeppen**. Chief Koeppen has been with the AHFD since 1980 and, as you might have guessed, he was also a paramedic. He comes from a large family where eight members are firemen or paramedics. His father was the first full-time fire chief in Wheeling, Illinois. He was with that department for forty-three years. The chief's older cousin, Ken Koeppen, from the Mt. Prospect Fire Department, was in the charter paramedic class.

Koeppen like most of his paramedic brethren appears to be a pretty laid back guy. Not physically imposing or impressive and, along the lines of Chief Loesch, a pretty average looking, middle class, white guy with a strong Chicago accent. Friendly, accommodating, and obviously competent, he pretty much sailed into the chief's job after a long, distinguished career as a paramedic who came up through the ranks of his department.

Characterizing his being named chief, as 'sailing in', is perhaps a bit inaccurate because in the incredible lineage of paramedic/firefighters that Zydlo trained, Ken Koeppen can be described as a second generation paramedic. He did not get on the job until eight years after the inaugural class. He is, however, a product of that excellence that all those first paramedics displayed and passed on to their subsequent partners and eventual replacements.

In the fire service, paramedics only remain in that position until they take a promotion into upper management. Once you obtain a higher supervisory role you are generally done with routine ambulance runs. Koeppen had left that role in the dust a long time ago---or at least he thought he had.

December 12, 2013
In the Belly of the Beast

"If anybody comes down here, that's it. Any tear gas, anything. I already shot a cop. I am not afraid to shoot her," Eric M. Anderson, 41, said in a chilling recording released by the Northwest Central Dispatch System.

Ken Koeppen was off duty, having dinner with his wife, at his father-in-law's home. It was a classic, cold, miserable day in the dead of another ball-busting Chicago winter. He and his father-in-law were settling in to watch TV when Ken noticed emergency lights across the street. He looked out the window and saw an empty squad car in the neighbor's driveway.

Arlington Heights veteran police officer Michael McEvoy (52) was having a routine shift until he ran into the very disagreeable Eric Anderson. McEvoy was dispatched to Anderson's girlfriend's house where Anderson had already shot one person. A 911 call to dispatch recorded some additional gunshots, so McEvoy knew the body count could rise rapidly. Consequently, he was first through the door and got shot down before he could get a shot off. He is out of the fight and to say the least, his chances for getting to mass at St. James on Sunday were not good.

But, Anderson was fixing to have an even worse day then McEvoy. He had, without any provocation or reason, shot a police officer at close range with a 9mm semi-automatic pistol. Officer McEvoy never had a chance. Although Anderson was known to be a pretty disagreeable asshole on a good day, his bad behavior had never reached this level.

Ken Koeppen had meandered over to the neighbor's residence without any clue of the drama occurring, when the cavalry came skidding up to the house where McEvoy was just starting to have the absolute worst frigging day of his life. McEvoy was on the kitchen floor with blood pumping out of his neck at Mach 1.

The police didn't hesitate. They charged into the kitchen, guns drawn. Anderson took off into another part of the house while the police dragged the unconscious and critically wounded McEvoy out of the house and started first aid. Koeppen, whose adrenaline was pounding and surging through his body, (remember just two minutes before he thought he was walking over to help with a probable busted hip or twisted ankle) now had a veteran cop at his feet whose life was flowing out onto the floor. A couple officers desperately tried to stop the bleeding.

Koeppen, who hasn't been on an ambulance in a very long time---eighteen years---doesn't blink. That old muscle memory, that Zydlo-based training, the repetitive actions of hundreds of emergency calls, just jump right off of Koeppen. He yells at his wife to get some bath towels. Koeppen who is fifty-three, (and let's face, it fifty-three is not thirty-three) just does what his training, his experience, his damn entire being dictates, he launches his ass onto McEvoy and does what he has done hundreds of times in thirty-three plus years on the job.

Koeppen leans into McEvoy's face and puts as much pressure on the wound as he can. The bleeding slowed. The troops arrived and put McEvoy into the ambo. They pull out all the stops, as they would do for anyone, but a cop is one of them and no one in the back of the ambo wants to go to a funeral and tell McEvoy's parents, "We tried our best, sorry." Nope. This is special on steroids and everyone knows it. No one has to say a word. Failure is not even a remote option.

Koeppen saved McEvoy's life and, of course, the other medical personnel did their jobs just like Dr. Zydlo drew it up. It worked, like it almost always does, in spite of Anderson's best efforts. That night, the machine hummed in a glory-filled, magnificent way, resulting in all kinds of amazing news.

The hostage standoff continued for a couple more hours and predictably there were more cops at the scene than strippers at a 1985 Chicago Bears' team party. The police were not in a forgiving mood, so Mr. Anderson's odds for seeing another sunrise were a long shot. Had Anderson suddenly decided he would rather be a hero at the penitentiary for the next several decades, he could have walked out, hands up, and survived. Even in Chicago, the police will generally not shoot you on live TV.

At around 10:30 pm., Anderson came out of the house, hostage in tow with a gun to her head, making a beeline for the garage. It seemed like a good plan until two SWAT guys stepped out of the shadows and lit Mr. Anderson up "after he pointed a gun at them." No need for the paramedics on this one. Mr. Anderson was apparently dead enough that nothing short of divine intervention would help him.

Mike McEvoy fully recovered and eventually went back to work.

Koeppen, the acting fire chief at the time of this particular event (the city was conducting a nationwide search for a new fire chief) was quickly and officially named the permanent fire chief and at least for a little while, the world was right.

Chief Koeppen received awards from every group in a hundred-mile radius for saving McEvoy's life. Meanwhile, the boys back at the fire house(s) were celebrating---like the Count of Monte Cristo at a debutante ball---their chief's heroics because every fireman in Arlington Heights had just gotten "a get out of jail free card" for the next twenty years or so.

Chief Ken Koeppen, like many of the paramedics before him, does what he does without thought of reward or glory. He does it simply because that is who he is and what he is about. Koeppen is just the sort of paramedic that Stan Zydlo imagined when he was dreaming up this concept. "Keep it simple. Do what you have to do to save them. Stabilize them, transport them, and hope the ER folks know what they are doing when your victim hits those emergency room doors."

In the grand, and now fairly distinguished and accomplished long history of the paramedics and their chiefs, Ken Koeppen joins a very exclusive, small group of paramedics who have come up from the bottom to become chief of their department. Perhaps, in the grand scheme of time, Ken Koeppen's actions will fade from everyone's memory. Maybe, by the time he retires, this heroic episode won't make the cut at his retirement ceremony. One thing is for certain, though, Ken Koeppen knows very deep down in the recesses of his heart that he may be a hot shit chief of a pretty big fire department, but at the core of his soul, he is first and foremost a *paramedic*.

Bruce Rodewald is a leader in every sense of the word. Even today after being retired for eleven years, he has that steely-eyed wolf look. If you have an ounce of common sense, you understand really quick that this seemingly old dude is not to be trifled with. He is former U.S. Army Chief Warrant Officer who flew hundreds of combat missions as a Huey pilot during two tours in Vietnam. When you experience the entire Soviet military armament being thrown at your ass every day for two of the bloodiest years of the war (1966-1968), everything after that is pretty much gravy. So after being discharged and waiting for a job with TWA to fly passenger jets, Rodewald was approached by a family friend who suggested that he might like working as a fireman in his hometown of Arlington Heights, Illinois.

Rodewald was lukewarm about it ("Shit, let's see standing on the back of a fire truck in December freezing my nuts off or flying a 727 with hot stewardesses hanging around") he took the test and the rest is history. He was hired in March of 1971, and predictably as his typical talent and moxie had a habit of doing, he pretty much raced through the ranks at Mach I.

After just eight years on the job (July of 1978) he was a lieutenant. Five years later, in September of 1983, he was a captain. Less than a year later, in May of 1984, he was the chief of Chicago's largest suburban fire department. At 38 years old, he was the youngest chief of a major fire department in the United States. He had reached the top in record-breaking speed and it didn't take him long to wonder, "What the fuck did I get myself into?"

Chief Rodewald was not one of the original founding fire chiefs of the EMS/Paramedic Program, but he was, without question, a critical player in modernizing and bringing his fire department kicking and screaming into the twentieth century. He was the bridge between old school, good old boy fire service and the new modern lean and mean professional fire service. He quickly found out that fighting a hundred years of bad tradition would, on some days, make gun fights with Charlie over Vietnam look like Romper Room.

It, of course, started with the simplest of personnel decisions. Rodewald knew it was coming and he knew there would be resistance. It was time to bring women into the fold and allow them to be firefighters as long as they passed the required tests and were qualified. Arlington Heights is an upper middle class suburb. Many of the then 77,000 residents were well-educated and successful. Hiring women was news, but it wasn't a hot button event---unless you were a fireman.

Rodewald had his way, but the line in the sand was drawn. Rodewald was now officially "management" and the gap between him and his firemen was permanent. So be it. Someone had to lead and someone had to do the job. He understood this. He was not shy and did not get skittish when a confrontation brewed. He was right in the middle of this huge transition period in the fire service.

After years of general neglect, his department's equipment was broken down and in bad shape. The firehouses were old, unsafe and dilapidated. Training was inadequate. He inherited supervisors who were riding out their time until retirement. He had young guys coming up "who got it". He had to juggle running chainsaws to modernize and get the department up to standard.

None of this was fun. He served at the pleasure of the city manager a "professional" hired by the mayor and board of trustees to manage the day-to-day operations of the village, town, or city. During his tenure as chief, he would work for five acting, or elected, mayors and three city managers. Each of them had someone else they would like to make fire chief, but none of them had the nerve to do it. None, with the exception of City Manager Ken Bonder (who originally hired Rodewald), had the warm fuzziest towards the chief, but neither did they want to screw with their most dynamic and charismatic department head. Rodewald was not a Rhodes Scholar. He was street smart and had those special leadership chops. He set goals and accomplished them. He did not like hearing the word "No". He'd get a major project done and move onto the next one. He expected and demanded excellence from everyone. The high-level performers loved him because he stayed out of their way and gave them a lot of autonomy and support. If you were a problem child, he'd light your ass up. No, the Chief did not play and the thing about it was that it worked. Even his detractors saw the changes. Often he dragged them by the heels to the next goal, but eventually it was all good and the fire department got more professional by the day.

He was the eye of the storm and that was the way he liked it. He never asked anyone to do anything he would not do. He'd get dirty in a minute. There was not a prima donna bone in him.

Dr. Zydlo knew Rodewald and had seen him around for years, but it wasn't until he was made chief that they bonded and became close. Rodewald understood and absolutely saw the way of the future for fire departments. It would not be fighting fires. Already this whole paramedic thing was becoming the primary mission of the department. The old timers hated the idea, but the fact was houses were no longer burning down with any regularity. It was EMS and EMS was the way of the future.

Rodewald and Zydlo got each other. Both former professional soldiers, they knew who each other was, where they were each coming from, and what needed to be done. They were both loyal and honest to a fault. These two alpha males made shit happen quickly.

They were about as subtle as a twenty-pound sledgehammer. They had similar styles of "my way or the highway". They both hated politicians and all the negative connotations that came with that. They each knew that they would not win any popularity contests. Frankly, they didn't give a shit either. If they were in a meeting and working together, they would run over the opposition. They were kindred spirits and often in that same foxhole. They were as is said today, "brothers from a different mother".

Zydlo watched Rodewald almost double the number of paramedics in Arlington Heights. When he first became chief, there were around thirty paramedics. When he left, there were over fifty and every fireman was at least an EMT. Rodewald led the charge for the latest and greatest equipment. All of this had a ripple effect on the other fire departments. The modernization of the paramedics and the significant increase in funding had the desired effect of saving more lives. Dr. Zydlo thought that Chief

Rodewald was yet another turning point in the growth and prominence of the EMS system. Like Zydlo, Rodewald read the tea leaves well.

It was August 1, 1985 and Rodewald had been Chief for about 15 months when Arlington Park Race Track caught on fire. Arlington Park had been in business for 58 years at that point. Like all older racetracks it was a frigging tinderbox. In spite of Rodewald's efforts of strict fire code enforcement, the racetrack was old, really old and its owner was the single, biggest taxpayer in Arlington Heights. This operation, which was seasonal, brought in tens of millions of dollars into the local economy. This was a pretty big deal and it was Rodewald's largest property disaster during his tenure as chief.

The fire started around 2:15 am and quickly got out of control. The entire fire department responded and fought the fire for over 24 hours. Rodewald didn't go to bed or home for three days. At least twenty-two fire departments responded and over two hundred firefighters fought the fire for at least twelve hours. Rodewald had all the help and expert advice he could ever need, including two senior Chicago Fire Chiefs who were on scene and offering assistance. Rodewald asked them to do a quick inspection and offer an opinion as to what else could be done. After about a half hour they returned and one of the chiefs said to Rodewald, "Well Chief, you could drop this son of a bitch into Lake Michigan and it wouldn't matter."

They successfully fought the fire without any loss of life. No horses died and his firemen worked like animals to contain and make sure that the fire didn't spread any further. As always, there were a lot of lessons learned, and protocols and SOPs were tweaked in the aftermath. All in all, not a horrible experience for all concerned. Everyone, except Chief Rodewald. The local paper was outraged. They were pissed and this whole disaster had to be somebody's fault, right? They were not about to attack one of their biggest advertisers (the racetrack), so the Chief quickly became the whipping boy.

By golly, by gosh, why didn't the fire department prevent the fire? Where were all the fire code violations that should have been enforced by the Chief? Does the Chief know how much money this would cost the city in lost revenue? What they really meant to say was "Does he realize how much lost revenue the paper would sustain in lost advertising"? No, the gloves were off and they decided that they would make an example of Rodewald.

Chief Rodewald, who didn't much care for the media in general, really got a case of red ass. "Are these guys serious? This is my fault?"

Rodewald, who isn't exactly known for his gregarious sense of humor, was red, fucking hot. To add additional insult, the goofy politicians, who very seldom even thought about the fire department, were all becoming firefighting experts.

The racetrack owners were not the least bit upset. They had wisely invested in all sorts of insurance policies. One of those policies covered "Loss of income". Another covered "Current replacement value"; yet another "Business interruption". Nope, old Arlington Park might be history, but the new racetrack would become the biggest and most beautiful track ever constructed in the horse racing industry. Not only that, but the experts placed the property damage at twenty- two million dollars. The racetrack owners and their attorneys would eventually wrangle seventy-five million out of the insurance companies. The insurance companies might not have been too happy, but the racetrack folks were absolutely giddy with the end result.

Rodewald survived the attack on him when cooler heads prevailed and everyone quit paying attention to the scandalous, yet unproven and undocumented headlines. He had been contemplating retirement, but decided to stay on as Chief. He wound up being the longest serving Chief in his department's history. At the time he retired, he had served as Chief for over twenty years and his department was rated Class One, up from the Class Three rating when he was named Chief. After he left, they were downgraded to a Class Two.

Finally, in the category of six degrees of separation,[2] the Chief's wife, Nancy (nee Scanlon) Rodewald was a twelve-year-old girl on December 1, 1958 when the Our Lady of the Angels' fire broke out, killing 92 students. On that day Nancy was in the fifth grade in Sister Mary St. Canice's class at Our Lady of the Angels. Fortunately, she was one of the lucky ones. She and Bruce had two sons and, as you might guess, they are also firemen and paramedics. Does anyone wonder what the grandchildren will do for a living?

CHAPTER SIX

Profane Eloquence

"When I want my men to remember something important, to really make it stick, I give it to them double dirty. It may not sound nice to some bunch of little old ladies at afternoon tea party, but it helps my soldiers to remember. You can't run an army without profanity and it has to be eloquent profanity. An army without profanity could not fight its way out of a piss soaked paper bag... As for comments I make sometimes I just, By God get carried away with my own eloquence".
– General George S. Patton

L͟ike most of the early paramedics, Zydlo was a veteran. In the world of alpha males, this is a pretty big deal due to the fact that only 7.3 percent of all Americans have served in the military.[3] That is a very exclusive club and, in alpha male circles, it is almost mandatory in order to be taken seriously. Certainly, it is mandatory if one wished to lead because former soldiers, marines, airmen and naval personnel know and respond to quality leadership that comes from their fraternity. Any attempt to lead by someone who does not possess these abilities generally does not end well.

In Stan's case, his bona fides were intact. As a former Air Force Captain who was a flight surgeon, Stan spoke the language. He was not a member of the firefighter community, but he was a vet and that was the next best thing. Stan's initial assignment in the USAF was at the School of Aerospace Medicine at Brooks Air Force base in San Antonio, Texas.

After that, he was assigned to Blytheville Air Force Base in Blytheville, Arkansas. For the next two years, he flew on top secret nuclear B-52 flights over the former Soviet Union. After two years of active duty, he transitioned into the Air Force Reserve where he was assigned to Bunker Hill Air Force Base, later known as Grissom AFB, in Indiana.

As with everything in Stan's life, this was a great learning experience. The military, for all its great attributes, is just like any other well-funded, organized community. There are politics, jealousies, job jockeying, and all manner of human drama playing out on a daily basis. As far as he was concerned, it was all one big learning experience to absorb and build upon.

Certainly, Stan was an experienced medical professional at this point. He was just finishing a stint as an Air Force Flight Surgeon when fate called him to a small, Indiana town.

Wabash, Indiana is famous for exactly nothing. Located in the center of Indiana, the population hovers around 10,000. It is the quintessential, small American town made up of a well-educated middle class. In 1964, Wabash had something most cities that size did not---a great medical doctor who could do it all.

Dr. Carl Elward had no issues with being a small town doctor. He understood and realized that he had few equals when it came to medical knowledge. The challenges were, well, challenging. There was no large urban hospital teaching center close by. You sank or swam on your own guts and talent. He preferred it that way. The fewer bureaucrats he had to deal with, the better he liked it. He liked being the final authority and his new protégé liked it better than he did.

Elward also knew that specialists be damned, he could do his and their job better than they could most of the time. He was not only good; he was goddamn brilliant. He and his partners knew it. He was the classic small town doctor who had been around long enough that he not only probably delivered you when you were born, but he would also be there when you died.

So when the younger and bolder Dr. Stanley Zydlo, Jr. showed up in 1964, Carl knew he had a handful to deal with. It was clear that Stan was exceptionally bright. Carl had no doubt that Stan was something special. The problem would be to corral all this energy. Stan could go non-stop for days.

Arriving in Wabash with a wife and four kids, Stan was ready to settle down. This was not exactly his idea of cutting edge, high drama medicine, but he would not only make lemonade when handed lemons, he would turn it into vodka and lemonade and have a party. But Wabash, Indiana was about as culturally far away from his hometown of Chicago as was Brazil. Once again, Stan found himself in a small town, rural situation. He felt exiled into the proverbial boonies.

It was here in Wabash that Zydlo felt like he "learned to be a real doctor." Even after practicing medicine for over fifty years, he considered Dr. Elward "the finest physician I ever saw or worked for. Without question, Elward was the most complete and qualified physician I ever saw."

While working for Dr. Elward, Zydlo learned to care for any and all patients who came to their office and also to respond to the Wabash County emergency room when their patients went there.

Stan was up to his neck immediately. Having joined the Air Force right out of medical school, he did no residencies anywhere and thus, had no specific expertise. He worked on pediatric, orthopedic, gynecological, obstetrical, and geriatric cases, as well as administering anesthesia or assisting in general surgeries.

Zydlo and Elward also performed complicated neurological procedures and surgeries. There was nothing Dr. Elward was afraid to tackle and Zydlo thought that the on-the-job training he received with Elward was world class. Many years later, he would understand and appreciate what a medical savant Elward was. If you could ask Dr. Zydlo who was the best doctor he ever saw, he would tell you, "without question, Carl Elward."

In Wabash, there were no board certified doctors in any specialty. They were all general practitioners. If someone got sick beyond the capabilities of Drs. Elward and Zydlo, they were sent to Ft. Wayne, Indiana (47 miles away), or to Marion, Indiana (22 miles away). A registered nurse ran the emergency room that they utilized. There was no doctor in the ER. People came by themselves, or were brought to the ER by friends or relatives. There were no ER docs or ambulances. Comparing today's ER with those of mid-1960s was like comparing 1960s medicine to 1860s medicine.

Zydlo would later reflect back on those days and understand just how talented the rural physicians were. Their results were almost always good, and the community they worked in appreciated their often super-human efforts. Wabash proved to be a great training ground for what was to come in Stan Zydlo's life.

After working four years in Wabash, Dr. Elward decided to leave to go into a radiology residency. That left Stan with a huge medical practice. In addition to doing this work, Stan had married while attending medical school, and the youngest of their four children was severely disabled. He and a friend built a home for 150 disadvantaged children in Wabash, another in Watch Park, Illinois (near Rockford) and one in Peru, Indiana. Coupled with these ever busier homes for disabled children, and USAF reserve duties, Stan was never home. Consequently, his marriage broke down and his wife returned to her hometown of Kansas City with the children.

Stan had been away from Chicago for a very long time at this point, but it never failed to call him home. It is difficult to explain to people, but most Chicagoans have a love-hate relationship with the city. There is no other place like it. The city has a soul, a certain rhythm to it. If we were able to remove the politicians and violence from it, it could be almost perfect, save the shitty winters.

It was around this time that Zydlo read about a group of physicians who were developing an emergency medical specialty to staff emergency rooms. There were also efforts of a small group of physicians in Michigan attempting to put together a residency program for emergency medicine. This was around 1968, so right in line with the Zydlo sweet spot.

Stan knew his tendency to dive in at a hundred miles per hour had helped destroy his marriage. He was not thinking along the lines of a relatively set work schedule, time off, no fee collecting problems, no staff or office expenses, and, of course, no malpractice insurance costs. Couple that with a comprehensive on-call specialty roster to confer with and this was shaping up to be a dream job.

Stan being Stan, located the Medical Emergency Service Associates (MESA) in Chicago. MESA provided a group that staffed emergency rooms for Chicago area hospitals. He called, got an appointment with the president who was also a physician, and was hired on the spot. So began the phase of his life that would change the way medicine and prehospital care was practiced worldwide.

In 1969, Zydlo went to work at MESA and was assigned to Northwest Community Hospital in Arlington Heights. When he arrived, the emergency room received about 10,000 patients per year. Due to the huge population shift and migration from Chicago, it soon grew to 20,000 patients a year.

There were no nearby hospitals to the west or north, but there were major highways all around Northwest Community which made it well-positioned to receive the ever increasing trauma victims from automobile accidents and reckless activities at the ever increasing number of bars. Add on the everyday pedestrian home accidents, cardiac events and other medical emergencies and Northwest Community quickly became one of the bigger players in the hospital business.

When Zydlo arrived at Northwest Community, there were exactly two private ambulance companies who brought patients to the ER. None of the personnel knew anything beyond basic Red Cross First Aid. Trauma victims were lucky to get a Kotex pad slapped on a bleeding wound. Zydlo was often on the receiving end of all this drama and truly felt sorry for both the victims and the ambulance personnel who were untrained and pretty much helpless.

Now was the time. He knew it, but there was no curriculum. No videos. No Power Points, Nada. He had no heavenly idea on what or how, but it was going to happen---right now---and that was the end of that. One small issue would be the actual time. Where in the hell was the time going to come from to do all these things? How do you reinvent the wheel in your spare time? Oh yeah…and who would fund this little project? For that matter, who would draw up and type all the course materials? What about the logistics? Just figuring out the mundane and boring was a nightmare.

Finally, he just had to say fuck it and wing it until he made it because if he didn't, the program was not going to happen. It was just too overwhelming and burdensome. When Zydlo really considered all of it, he didn't wonder why no one had attempted to put together a modern paramedic and emergency medical services system on the scale that he envisioned. This was an absolute first and the pure, unadulterated gall of thinking that he could pull it off burned the ass of every bureaucrat and naysayer within an earthquake's distance.

In life, timing is everything. Can you imagine the field day naysayers could have had if the internet was available in 1969 and every asshole with a computer could have weighed in anonymously on the subject? They would have strung Zydlo and the firemen up. The program would have died before the first class and millions more would have died unnecessarily. No, the timing was perfect. All Zydlo had to do was make it happen. No problem.

Well, it was not a problem as long as he didn't think about what had to be done and here is where Dr. Zydlo glowed. He was able to compartmentalize every aspect of what he had planned, very much like he practiced medicine in an emergency room. Before he could do step three or four, he had to do step one and two. Step three or four may be the big long-term issue, but if step one (keeping the patient breathing) was not attended to immediately, he would never get to step four. For example, he knew without question, that if the law as it stood was not radically and completely changed, it did not matter how many firemen he trained.

Nevertheless, he put that little issue aside and concentrated on training the soon-to-be heroes. This was all very much like the space program. Initially, everyone at NASA had scoffed at the idea of putting a human in space. Chimpanzees were the choice of the NASA scientists. Pilots? Those arrogant fighter jocks? Are you crazy? The chimps were just as smart and served the same purpose. Why would we put up with those prima donna pilots?

Why indeed? Zydlo's issues with his colleagues, the nurses, and political clout were much the same dynamic at play as those at NASA. The scientists (the doctors) hated the whole paramedic idea. "By God, it will ruin medicine. It will diminish our role as medical professionals."

The firemen (astronauts) were of the opinion that "Hey, we keep you breathing until we get you to Zydlo. What's the problem?"

Forty plus years later, we all now know what Dr. Zydlo instinctively knew then---that firemen, like their brethren at NASA, absolutely had the "right stuff."

CHAPTER SEVEN

And...So It Began

"The task of leadership is not to put greatness into people,
But to elicit it, for the greatness is there already."
–John Buchan

Standing in front of two hundred and eight firemen in a bare bones fire department bay, Dr. Stanley Zydlo, Jr. was a man in full. This was simply his destiny. This was what he was born for and yet, as he stood there what he was about to do was totally and completely against the law. Additionally, he was an alpha male in a roomful of ultra, alpha males who literally ran into burning buildings that were exploding and collapsing on top of them. They had one thing in common and that was, to a man, they were fearless, with an attitude of, "If you can do it, so can I."

What Zydlo was about to do had never been attempted before. No one gave this any chance of succeeding and, on top of that, Zydlo had the entire medical profession hoping and praying that he would fail. These were powerful enemies. As Zydlo stood there, he wasn't even getting paid. So, in addition to breaking the law, he was doing it for free. Still, he had no doubts. This was the right thing at the right time and anyone who didn't like it could go fuck himself.

The firemen sat dead still, waiting for something profound to happen. Outside of Stan, nobody had a clue as to what would occur in the next few months. Zydlo looked out at this motley, undisciplined, tough guy, take no prisoners gang and thought to himself, "I cannot bullshit or trifle with this group. I am going to have to kick them in the balls to get their attention and then hold it. If they think I'm lying, bullshitting, or manipulating them for one second, I will lose them." He had no intention of doing any of those things, but he knew how critical these first hours, and few days, would be.

What he was about to do had never been attempted outside of a medical school. These were not men who had prepared for years and years to gain admittance into a world class, advanced medical studies program. These cats, for the most part were lucky to have graduated high school without a felony arrest. These were the guys the mothers of girls had warned them about since puberty. Still they had a quiet confidence about them, an eagerness to prove themselves. They had been doing stuff their entire lives that other people were afraid to do. They had a trait, a genetic quality that was valued in every walk of life and every society. They were fearless and had a perpetual chip on their shoulders.

These dudes were warriors in every sense of the word. In their hearts and minds there was nothing that you could do to break them. Whatever you threw at them they could handle. This Zydlo guy, what could he do to them? They ate guys like him for breakfast. A lot of them didn't want to be there, goddammit, they were *firefighters*. Who wants to put Band-Aids on some spoiled rich brat in Inverness? Worse yet, who wants to haul some 350-pound fat ass out of a fourth floor apartment building on a stretcher meant to carry a 180-pound guy?

So, with no one except Dr. Zydlo having any idea what was going to happen or how it would play out short or long term, the first semi-formal, non-sanctioned, unlicensed, unsupervised illegal paramedic instruction class was about to start at the Mt. Prospect Fire Department in suburban Chicago. Stan Zydlo had everyone exactly where he wanted them, dazed and confused.

He had little trouble getting their attention with his opening salvo. Standing in front of the room to introduce himself, Zydlo picked up a 20-gauge needle attached to a bag of IV saline solution, hung the bag on a nail on a post and rammed that one inch needle up the main vein on the back of his left hand while the firemen sat in stunned silence.

No one breathed. No one spoke, some recall thinking, "Did that crazy fucker just stick that big ass needle into his hand?"

They had all seen it, just couldn't believe it. They continued to sit in stunned silence while Zydlo explained the importance of getting liquids into every trauma victim. Zydlo wasn't sure if they were listening because they all stared at his hands, their mouths wide open. They didn't quit staring until he said, "Tomorrow, all of you are going to take this 20-qauge needle and stick it in your partner's hand."

"What, what did he just say?" "Is he frigging crazy?" "He can kiss my ass, isn't nobody sticking me with anything."

In his next breath, Zydlo said, "If any of you think you are not going to do this, pack your shit up and get out."

No one moved and thus the whole tone was set for the next several weeks. By the end of the course, the backs of their hands looked like pincushions.

The one thing Stan had going for him with the firemen was that they all realized very quickly that because of his medical knowledge and the subject matter that alone caused him to stratospherically outrank them. In a quasi-military environment this helps a great deal. It also didn't hurt that Stan was a former Air Force Captain, Golden Gloves boxing champion, street fighter and all around light weight badass who, when all else failed, *would* step into the alley and work it out. All of this was always percolating below the surface, so it took a few days for everyone to measure their dicks and sort it out.

But, sort it out they did and things soon settled down. Basically, it went something like this: "Anyone who doesn't want to be here...leave." "Anyone who does not want to follow my directions exactly as I teach them...leave." "Anyone who does not think they can stick their face in a pile of steaming, bleeding guts and grab hold of it to stop the bleeding and save a life should get out...now."

The firemen were thinking "We aren't at the Waffle House now. This fucker is crazy."

Collectively, none of them had ever heard a medical professional talk like this. A doctor? A crazy one at that. They all thought, "let's stick around and see how this plays out."

While Zydlo thought, "All right. I have these crazy bastards right where I want them."

Zydlo found a rhythm and discovered very quickly that these guys were good. They were quick, smart and like sponges. If he had enough time, he could start teaching them open heart surgery. He fell in love with the group because they were even more trainable than he, or anyone else, would have guessed. On an intellectual level, this was shocking to most. Zydlo thought he had struck gold. None of these men had the natural, God-given talent that he had. He knew it---and they knew it. What was so surprising was that they had the capacity to figure it out. It did not matter now complicated or how technical the issue was. They learned stuff that was taught on an advanced level in medical school.

Zydlo loved to tease and test them. He loved to watch them compete with one another. He would walk in to class and say something like, "Ok, what was the name of the lead elephant in Hannibal's caravan when the Carthaginians crossed the Alps to invade Italy?"[4] The boys thought, "What? What did that asshole just ask us?" Zydlo would just switch back to a normal medical subject and continue on as if that was a perfectly normal question to ask.

There was a purpose to the madness, however. He wanted the guys to handle anything that was thrown at them. If they didn't know the answer, they had better figure it out quickly. It did not matter that it had nothing to do with the subject matter. It was an intellectual exercise to get them thinking outside the box. It was another way to figure out difficult problems. It was an old military trick used to teach leadership. It was effective because the men did not question the reason the question was asked. They understood one thing---they had better have the answer tomorrow.

Local librarians were at a loss to explain the sudden, almost daily, appearances of uniformed firemen hanging out in the reference section of the library. But one thing was certain. By the next class everyone knew the name of the elephant and the history behind it. No one had a clue as to why this was important, but Zydlo knew and he could not have been more pleased. His boys were doing far more than anyone would have guessed.

No matter what happened next, political pressure, non-believing doctors and medical community, they were isolated, on an island alone. It was Zydlo and the soon to be paramedics. Zydlo was making them his tribe. These were his guys, goddammit, and nobody better think they were going to fuck around with them. If they tried, he would eviscerate their asses.

Zydlo took care of his tribe. He provided security, love, belonging, self-esteem and an understanding of their place in the world. He offered them everything they could want in this world. Ground Zero was the paramedics. Behind them stood Dr. Stanley Zydlo. This combination would prove to be undefeatable.

In the initial group, fifty of the 208 men were there on their own time. The inaugural class training was two to three hours each, four days a week during evening hours for a total of 58.5 hours. That was basically the EMT class.

Classes were held in the fire departments of Arlington Heights Station Number 2, Mt. Prospect's main station, Hoffman Estates Station Number 1 on Saturdays and the Palatine Fire Department station on Sundays. Seven to ten hours were held at Northwest Community Hospital, and even the occasional class in Dr. Zydlo's garage at home.

The Advanced Paramedic course encompassed a 234-hour course with a cost of $25.00. Sometimes the paramedic candidates paid for the course out of their own pockets. Today it is a whole different story. Starting with the money, alone, the breakdown and numbers are astronomical. However, before delving into the economic issues, consider this. In the inaugural course, 208 signed up or were volunteered. Out of those 208 men, 186 went on to the Paramedic course.

After another 234 hours of instruction, 186 men took the test. 107 passed. That's it---*107.* That was the inaugural, first ever group of Paramedics. From that class, a medical and financial juggernaut was born. Prior to the 107 men who graduated this course, there were *no* Paramedics. *Zero.*

Today, or at least in the records from 2012, the State of Illinois reported 22,398 licensed EMTs and 13,956 licensed Paramedics. All fifty states have stringent licensing requirements. The Bureau of Labor Statistics reported, in 2012, that there were 239,100 licensed paramedics. The forecast at least an additional 55,000 paramedics by 2022. It is almost certain that in 1972, no one could have predicted this when Dr. Zydlo trained those initial 107 paramedics.

It now takes almost two years to train a paramedic with about 1,000 hours of classroom time. There are half a dozen interviews, drug screen tests, at least $7,500 in associated costs. That is in addition to annual licensing fees and continuing education. Consider for a moment what Dr. Zydlo did to train his guys and what the state now requires.

Are today's paramedic's better than those first classes? Are they better trained? They are certainly more regulated. Back then, it was Zydlo who made the rules. It was Zydlo who decided who would get yanked off the street. It was Zydlo who disciplined and trained them. In addition, Zydlo answered to no one. Eventually, all of that changed. The state started licensing everybody. Rules and regulations were piled on by the volume. Some were necessary, some chicken shit. It didn't matter---at some point, everything changes.

A few generations and several thousands of paramedics later, there is no right answer. It is akin to the old baseball/football/basketball argument. Was Oscar Robertson, who routinely average a triple double for a season better than Michael Jordan who never threw up a stat like that? Doubtful, but the stats would suggest otherwise. Was Babe Ruth better than Barry Bonds? Well, Baby played half-drunk most of the time and Barry was alleged to be a connoisseur of anabolic steroids and human growth hormones. Barry's stats are better, but, hell, Babe did play hung over on a regular basis. Finally, you have the old paramedics who did great things, really miraculous feats with little or no support. Their training was absolutely less than what is given today. Their support and equipment weren't even close to what is given today. Yet, once again, the old timers got it done and they got it done in creative and magnificent ways. In the final analysis, it does not matter.

The Dr. Zydlo course could have been called "Gunslinger Medicine, how to practice it without killing the patient." Dr. Zydlo was the ultimate Gunslinger. When it came to saving lives in hectic and high pressure situations, Zydlo had few peers. He had close to photographic memory. Once he committed himself to anything, it was an all-out effort on his part. He left no stones unturned and his effort was always far above and beyond what was called for.

For him, emergency medicine was simple. It was problem solving 101 at its most basic elements. First, do no harm. Second, stop the bleeding. Third, clear the airway. Fourth, treat for shock. The key to this whole paramedic business was to get the firemen to believe in themselves and to believe in Dr. Zydlo.

For the first few years, Zydlo's was pretty much the only voice they heard on the other end of the radio. The paramedics were, in fact and deed, Zydlo's eyes and hands in the street. This is what he had to get through the firemen's heads. This was the critical piece that had to happen for this to succeed. It was an easy statement to make. On the surface it sounds simple enough, but Zydlo was dead serious. This was exactly what he meant.

The firemen heard this over and over again, but it really didn't settle in until they were in the street administering to the sick and wounded. Zydlo would scream at them to do this or that without deviation or freelancing. The reasoning wasn't that Zydlo thought they were idiots or inadequate, but quite the contrary, if a problem arose, he wanted to take the responsibility. He believed he was far better equipped to "take the heat" if a mistake was made. When presented with the real world consequences, the firemen understood this. They finally "got it". Those who didn't got launched quickly.

As time progressed, the firemen were certain of two things: First and foremost, they better do exactly as Dr. Zydlo instructed them. No deviations, no debates, no second guessing. Second, they were in absolute fear of receiving a phone call the next day or after their shift from Dr. Zydlo. That meant one thing---they were in trouble and exactly how much depended on a number of factors. Occasionally, it only meant the Dr. Zydlo simply wanted to review what had happened on a particular call. If that were the case, everything was OK.

But if you somehow managed to screw up, lookout. Bad shit was about to rain down upon you. Zydlo simply did not care about hurt feelings, getting embarrassed, or looking bad in front of your peers. He would drag you into the ER and force you to reenact your actions that brought you in for a review. "The Review," as it became known, was not something you wanted to experience too often.

In today's world, Zydlo would not exist. There is not a chance in hell that he, or anyone else could create or start a program as far ranging as the paramedic profession. The odds that someone with Stan Zydlo's brains and moxie dropping down amongst us mere mortals are overwhelming. The mere thought of going against your superiors, your peers, the law, is so remote in today's political correctness environment, it simply would not happen.

The Inaugural, Charter Paramedic Class
"The First Evers"
December 1, 1972

Arlington Heights Fire Department

1. John Benson
2. Arthur R. Christenson
3. Gerald C. Collignon
4. Gerald C. Cullens
5. Robert L. D'Alberto
6. William G. Dressel
7. Edward C. Fitch, Sr.
8. Richard A. Frost
9. Dennis J. Horcher
10. Dennis L. Maihack
11. Gerald W. Nering
12. Dennis E. Ritter
13. Grover C. Rushing
14. William L. Spung
15. Craig R. Weidder

Buffalo Grove Fire Department

16. Clifford E. Burmeister
17. Robert A. Douglas
18. Ronald F. Ericksen
19. James A. Hansen
20. Eyrie S. Hilton
21. John Klbecka, Jr.
22. Arnold F. Krause, Jr.

23. Robert E. Krause
24. Ronald I. Olsen
25. Dominic J. Saviano, Jr.
26. Leslie W. Swieca
27. Joseph G. Wieser
28. Wayne L. Winter

Elk Grove Fire Department

29. John Pilkington
30. Larry Ryan
31. Gregg Riddle
32. Clyde Hood

Hoffman Estates Fire Protection District Number 1

33. David J. Baird, Jr.
34. David A. Farr
35. Charles J. Forton
36. Charles W. Fricke
37. David Gardner
38. Edward N. Kalasa
39. Richard A. Knapik
40. Joseph E. Minucciani
41. Gerald Nering
42. Joseph F. Nikrant
43. Terrence P. O'Callahan
44. Francis J. O'Shea
45. Francis J. O'Shea, Jr.
46. Patrick J. O'Shea
47. Thomas W. Ryan

48. Richard Weyker

Lake Zurich Police Department

49. William Cochrane
50. Paul Thiebault

Morton Grove Fire Department

51. Patrick J. Dunn
52. Albert G. Pitts
53. Donald Warner
54. Alan Weinstein

Mount Prospect Fire Department

55. Donald E. Barra
56. Arthur H. Boesche
57. William F. Brelle
58. Robert B. Clark
59. George T. Cullens
60. Lowell J. Fell
61. Arthur W. Felski
62. Charles J. Forton
63. John A. Gibson
64. Kenneth J. Koeppen
65. Robert D. Kooiker
66. Donald P. Reynolds
67. Kenneth B. Stahl
68. Ervin H. Villie

69. Richard Vincenzo
70. Paul Watkins
71. Leslie H. Wuollett

Palatine Fire Department

72. John E. Busch
73. Vernon Colie
74. William H. DePue
75. Richard H. Freeman
76. Barney Langer
77. William Noland, Jr.
78. James M. Ohlrich
79. George Palmer
80. Joseph F. Pannhausen
81. Huber Paske
82. Roy F. Wente
83. John Wente
84. John Wilson

Prospect Heights Fire Department

85. Gerald R. Glaser
86. Michael E. Pettingill
87. Randall F. Stephenson

Schaumburg Fire Department

88. John C. Dixon
89. Rolland G. Fitch

90. Richard Knapik
91. Donald R. Kopecky
92. James W. Naatz
93. Thomas P. Saltiel
94. Arthur W. Stoike

Rolling Meadows Fire Department

95. Bernard A. Abbink
96. Jack A. Anderson
97. Harold R. Bills
98. Paul W. Chybicki
99. Robert P. Cooney
100. Donald E. Gustafson
101. Roger L. Hugg
102. Theodore J. Loesch
103. Roger L. Mueller
104. William J. Palluck
105. William P. Schmidt
106. Charles W. Sellards

Waukegan Fire Department

107. William Rainey

CHAPTER EIGHT

The Paramedics

"Out of every one hundred men ten shouldn't even be there, eighty are just targets, nine are the real fighters, and we are lucky to have them, for they make the battle. Ah, but the one, one is a warrior, and he will bring the others back."
– Heraclitus, Greek Philosopher, 535 B.C. to 475 B.C

Nobody, and I mean nobody, knew how this whole paramedic thing would turn out. Stan Zydlo was going to turn loose a still unknown entity that would be highly trained and the best educated medical lifesaving apparatus known to man, and hand it over to a bunch of firemen. In less than six months, Zydlo taught 107 guys, who at the beginning could barely open a can of Band-Aids® without cutting themselves, into a mean, fast acting, incredibly complex, lifesaving group of over achievers who would be the core group of what would arguably become the most successful human lifesaving apparatus in the history of the western world.

He did this prior to a law being enacted by the Illinois legislature to make their activities legal. By July 13, 1972, he had the paramedics fully trained and ready to hit the streets. By October 1972, the law was enacted, but due to equipment and FCC issues they could operate until December 1, 1972.

The Northwest Suburban Emergency Medical Services began operations at 8 a.m. on December first. At 8:15 a.m., Buffalo Grove Paramedics Wayne Winter (who graduated first in the first paramedic class ever sanctioned and licensed) along with Dominic Saviano, Bob Krause and Robert Douglass saved the first life by performing advanced lifesaving techniques on a heart attack victim. Later that afternoon, Buffalo Grove Fire Department Paramedics saved a woman from choking to death. Zydlo and his paramedics never looked back.

The inaugural class break down by department/organization was as follows:

1.	Arlington Heights Fire Department	15
2.	Buffalo Grove Fire Department	13
3.	Elk Grove Village Fire Department	4
4.	Hoffman Estates Fire Department	16
5.	Lake Zurich Police Department	2
6.	Morton Grove Fire Department	4
7.	Mount Prospect Fire Department	17
8.	Palatine Fire Department 1	3
9.	Prospect Heights Fire Department	3
10.	Rolling Meadows Fire Department	12
11.	Schaumburg Fire Department	7
12.	Waukegan Fire Department	1

Total 107

From an initial class of 208 firemen who began training in May, 186 made it through the advanced emergency medical technician class. All of the paramedics and EMTs were Caucasian. They were all males. That first paramedic class graduated 107. The minimum passing score was 75%. Dr.

Zydlo was tough. Just less than 50% of the starting 208 made it to the paramedic level. Training was demanding and unforgiving. The only easy day was the day before. Daily it got more complicated, difficult, and challenging.

The paramedic candidates never knew what hit them. Remember, Zydlo walked into the class holding a bag of fluid and a big needle that looked like a weapon. He hung the bag on a nail, stuck the needle in the dorsal vein on the back of his left hand and started talking. The candidates stared at each other with a look that asked, "Who is this crazy bastard? Did he just stick that needle in his hand? Does he think *I'm* going to do that?"

Zydlo was a guided missile. There were no excuses allowed. You'd better be prepared, as you were required to stand in front of the class, give your answer, and defend your actions. The peer pressure mounted by the hour. Zydlo put them in a pressure cooker and watched them sweat. His constant refrain was, "You think it's tough in here, in a controlled and comfortable building? Well, wait until you are at an accident scene on a four lane highway, in the dark, in the snow, rain, and sleet, and people are bleeding to death because *you're a little uncomfortable.*" Zydlo drove these guys like Simon Legree with a whip. The firemen, just getting started, were shell-shocked. Who is this motherfucker?

Zydlo started with the basics. "We are in the lifesaving business here. It's a simple business. If you remember these three things we will save a lot of lives. First, we have to get oxygen to the body where it needs it. Second, you have to make sure there is enough blood in the system to carry that oxygen from the lungs to the other tissues in the body. Keep the blood inside the body. Last, make sure the airway is free of any obstruction so the lungs can do their job. This sounds really simple until you are doing all of this at a hectic pace, in a hostile neighborhood in the middle of a gang fight or another catastrophic event. The point is, it's always stressful and totally unpredictable."

Initially, the students were simply lost. Ninety percent of them were looking at this Dr. Zydlo dude who sounded like a doctor, looked like a doctor in his tie and short-sleeved white dress shirt, and pressed slacks, but he is a holy terror. There is no joking or fooling around, or charming this guy. He is an animal and he is scary.

When he looked at you with a laser like intensity and zero patience you just wanted to piss your pants. You're sitting there thinking, "God, don't let him call on me. Please look at someone else." The next thing you know you're standing up and he is firing questions at you. He's getting more pissed by the second. You're not answering quickly or correctly enough. He is raking your balls through hot coals. This is not much fun, and please tell me again why I volunteered to get terrorized by Dr. Crazy?

Zydlo didn't enjoy being a raging psychotic medical lunatic. He never did or said anything to which he hadn't given a great deal of thought. These fire and police men were an exceptional group for the most part. He knew exactly what kind of guy he needed. They had to have a high stress tolerance level, be able to adapt on the fly, be dependable, consistent, work as a team, have physical agility, and, most important, have common sense and an above average degree of intelligence.

After a few weeks they started to perform. The weak were weeded out or quit, and the bright ones excelled. He knew that putting them under high stress situations in the classroom world serve them well once they were on the street. He did not enjoy barking and biting at them. He wanted to be pals. These guys were funny, hardworking, and highly motivated--- his kind of guys, the type of company he preferred. However, there was so much at stake. If this program was not an immediate and overwhelming success it was dead in the water. These guys did not know it at the time, but their performance in the next weeks and months would be responsible for saving millions of lives in the decades to come.

Zydlo knew with every ounce of his being that this was a one shot deal. He and the firemen were in a foxhole. They were surrounded and few in the medical community wanted this program to succeed. Doctors and nurses, openly hostile, were the biggest obstacles. Zydlo realized that he had very little support outside of the fire chiefs, a few brave politicians, and his family.

Out of the bowels of hell and the Our Lady of the Angels Grammar School fire that stole and killed 92 children and three Roman Catholic nuns on December 1, 1958, the first official and state sanctioned paramedic program started fourteen years to the day of that disaster. As a young, medical student, Stan Zydlo watched helplessly as young kids dove out of windows onto the concrete. There were no paramedics or EMTs there to treat them. From December 1, 1972, through today, the presence of a highly trained and motivated paramedic service would always respond to any man made or natural disaster. They do it without exception and they do it without regard for their own personal wellbeing.

Most people cannot recall when there was not a highly-trained paramedic available 24/7. There were some attempts at training and responding to medical emergencies and accidents, but there was nothing even close to what Zydlo was putting together. There are a lot of people trying to take credit for this, but make no mistake---Dr. Zydlo and the Chicago Northwest Suburban departments listed here created and licensed the first real Paramedic/EMS system in the world.

The First Turnout

It was December 1, 1972, 0800hrs. and it was *go* day.

Stan and the 107 trained and now licensed paramedics were officially on the clock for the first time. There was no going back now. They would either kill people and this whole "paramedic thing" would die a quick death or they would, in fact, be the incredible and unbelievable juggernaut that would be responsible for saving millions of lives in the next forty-four years and beyond.

Dr. Stanley Zydlo, sitting in the ER at Northwest Community Hospital in Arlington Heights, Illinois, hovered over the radio gear waiting for the first call. The picture of a quiet, competent, professional, medical expert, he was, outwardly, his usual self-confident, Chuck Yeager type cool. Inwardly, he was boiling over. He had not slept in a week. His nerves were shot. He didn't have any idea who would catch the first tragedy. He was confident all his guys were good, but deep down he knew some of them were much better than others. He had trained and taught them, did everything in his power to clone their crazy ass selves in his own image. He had no doubt they would be the wolf pack he had nurtured and raised. Like any pack, the alpha male knew who was good, great or mediocre. He hoped the great ones would catch the first call.

Selling this thing was, in retrospect, marketing genius. Nobody wanted to buy it, rent it or marry it, but yet, "Here we are," Stan thought. "I just have no frigging idea what will happen."

The stress of those first moments would drop a fully grown horse. Zydlo's inclination was to jump in his car and cruise around hoping he would get to the first call, wherever that might be, and help out, or at least make sure no one got killed. He mentally dismissed that thought in a millisecond. He could do it, but he knew not to. No, his wolf pack would have to manage until they transported a patient to the emergency room.

It didn't take long to kick off. At 8:15 a.m. the first emergency paramedic call came into Buffalo Grove Fire Department and its all-volunteer paramedics. A huge siren went off in town and the men jumped into their privately-owned vehicles to race to the fire department and, from there, respond to the incident scene.

Dr. Zydlo was sitting at the hospital oblivious to all of this until the paramedics called it in. "Oh shit, a heart attack victim," he thought. He had hoped for something a little less serious, like a minor car accident, but, nope, they were starting at the top of the paramedic food chain. They had a seemingly healthy white female in full cardiac arrest on her living room sofa.

When Lt. Wayne Winter and Paramedics Dominic J. Saviano, Jr. and Robert Krause responded, Zydlo felt a little better because, as he put it many years later, Lt. Winter graduated at the top of the paramedic class. He was the ideal guy to catch the first ever paramedic call in the new system.

When the three men arrived at the victim's home, they were shocked to find fellow firefighter Bob Banderveir already there, but he was not on duty. It was his house and his young wife was the heart attack victim.

Winter, Saviano and Krause immediately started CPR and shocked her. She was revived and transported to Northwest Community Hospital where Dr. Zydlo treated her. She was eventually released to live a long life---a huge save for the future of EMS, a program that could have hung in the balance had they lost the victim.

The incident proved not to be a fluke because less than four hours later, the crew responded to an adult choking to death on a piece of food. The boys showed up and dislodged the food from the victim's windpipe, pulling off the second save of the young EMS system. Zydlo and his boys were in business and apparently business was going about as well as it could have gone.

Dominic Saviano is now eighty-three years old and has been retired from the Buffalo Grove Fire Department since 1995, a thirty-one-year career. He did thousands of calls, but he still recalls the first one with clarity. Dominic was your typical early paramedic: high school degree, raised on the west side of Chicago around Harrison and Kedzie, Army veteran of the Korean War, married with children. A former brick mason turned fire-fighter/paramedic, and ironies of ironies, his father, like Zydlo's father who was the owner of a neighborhood saloon, owned "Saviano's", a bar located on the west side.

When Saviano was interviewed, he explained that he and his colleagues did "just exactly what Dr. Zydlo taught us. We went through our protocol and we were able to save our friend's wife. At the time, we were certainly happy, but we really just did what Doc Zydlo taught us. It really wasn't that big a deal."

Who were these guys? For starters, perhaps the least bombastic and understated heroes ever put on this earth. Dominic Saviano could not be more humble if he had tried. Since 1959, he has lived in the same home with his wife, Joanne. They have been married for fifty-eight years, with three daughters and a son. They now have five grandchildren, and one great-grandchild, with another on the way. When they moved to Buffalo Grove in 1958, there were 708 residents. Today, there are almost 42,000.

Dominic is a first generation Italian-American. His father was a bricklayer/stonemason and tavern owner. His brothers were all bricklayers. He is a classic greatest generation guy and although his health declined with five stents in the arteries around his heart, a knee replacement, a hip replacement, a second hip replacement coming soon, he describes his health as excellent. You give Dominic Saviano a bag of lemons and he'll open a four-star restaurant.

That low key, lay low mentality of the pack was typical. The early paramedics felt the tension every time they hit the ER. The nurses initially hated all of them and most of the doctors were openly hostile. These conditions did not abate until a year or two into the program. By then, the paramedics were absolute rock stars. They were the princes of the city and they knew it. Most of them did not take advantage of their new found fame and recognition. Certainly, the family men like Saviano were most oblivious to it. However, there were some that *really* enjoyed the newfound legend status. There was even a nurse or two who really warmed up to the whole thing. All in all, this entire "paramedic thing" was virtually vibrating its way into the American psyche.

The Relentless Pressures

Even in death, Zydlo remains electrifying. He was the ultimate, uninsulated wire. The paramedics knew this, the medical establishment knew it, and he knew it. He had to temper his enthusiasm, as well as his temper, at every turn. He had zero doubt about what they were doing, but he also understood the very real and very powerful forces that did not and would not hesitate to do anything possible to see the program fail. This hummed along in the background for the first two years.

He kept this from everyone except Joyce, who would often bear the brunt of the stress and frustration that was never far away from Stan's entire existence. Joyce would say something like, "Stan, we have parent-teacher conferences next week. What day do you want to go?" Stan often would just say, "Goddammit, Joyce. I'm on call twenty-four-seven. You pick it."

This was the constant reply to almost any question involving scheduling, vacation, or anything that required planning. He hated himself for it and it mightily contributed to Stan's heart attacks, open heart surgeries, and the like. Joyce understood this and was very protective, as well as defensive, about Stan's unavailability to the point that she was almost grateful for a heart attack because that was the only thing that would slow him down for a few days. It actually took a catastrophic health event to slow Zydlo down. Outside of a few close confidants and Joyce, nobody had any idea of the physical and mental toll on him.

The old wolf knew and he knew what all alpha males know. If your enemies sense weakness, they will attack until they kill you. No, Stan never had any doubts about any of this. He never openly discussed it with the paramedics, but like their leader, they all had that wolf DNA, that sixth sense. It wasn't as defined as Stan's, but they developed it quickly. They lived it and now, because they were so vested in the program, they understood very quickly how this game was played. They were not happy and as time progresses, they got as defensive as their leader.

Stan saw that and appreciated it, but he had to nip it in the bud. He had problems enough and was well-equipped to deal with them. He saw it as part of his job. He had foreseen it long before the boys hit the street. He loved their loyalty, their willingness to throw down for him no matter who or what was the opposition. The wolf pack mentality was starting to take shape, was in the infant stage, but make no mistake about it, every successful run made the pack stronger and tighter.

The pressure that Dr. Zydlo put on his students was relentless. He was on them night and day, always within contact by radio. The radio was the lifeline. As the weeks and months progressed, the routine never varied. You'd go out on a call, evaluate the patient(s), start treatment and radio Zydlo. Saturday, Christmas Eve, whatever, he would pick up the radio and speak. It was like talking to the great Oz. If Stan was in the area of a bad accident or catastrophic event, he would show up, physically respond, and jump in. His actions never failed to impress his paramedics.

Forty-four years later, the surviving paramedics agree on one thing without exception: Dr. Zydlo was "The Man" in every respect. Bad accident on the side of a country road at three A.M., Zydlo showed up. A desperate mother watching her three-year-old choking to death on a Cracker Jack toy in a busy intersection, Zydlo showed up. Fire truck overturns on expressway and firemen critically injured, Zydlo showed up. This whole 'Forrest

Gump' existence is still mind boggling to the paramedics. The ER doctor on duty may respond, but Zydlo like the all-knowing, all-seeing Oz would dive in, in a millisecond if the ER doc said or instructed the paramedic to do something with which Zydlo disagreed. This did not endear him to his medical colleagues, but it sure did wonders for the esprit de corps of the paramedics.

As time went on and the paramedics became vastly more experienced, they would often bypass certain ER doctors on duty and contact Zydlo directly. On occasion, a serious pissing contest would escalate into a major beef because the paramedics would flat out refuse a medical order that they knew was inappropriate and or dangerous. Zydlo would be contacted and to his last day he could not recall when one of the paramedics was wrong. Much of this was because, at that time, there was not a specialty of 'emergency room physician'. Many of the doctors working the emergency room were regular internists, dermatologists etc. They simply did not have the requisite knowledge.

Make no mistake, Zydlo was as supportive as he could possibly be, but if a paramedic made a stupid mistake or failed to follow protocol, he would light him up. He lit them up on the radio. He lit them up in the ER if he was working. He was not quiet or shy about it.

As one paramedic stated, "Man, you did not want to fuck up and face the wrath of Dr. Z. Not a goddamn good thing would happen. He would drag you into the ER, his office, the parking lot, wherever. He would do it in front of everyone and anyone. If the offense were serious, he would not hesitate to yank your ass off the street."

He would work with you in the ER until he felt comfortable enough to put you back in the street. Never mind that you were employed by your fire department and Zydlo was employed by the hospital. In Zydlo's mind, you worked for him, period.

"Buddy, when your ass hit those emergency room doors you'd better be willing to check your ego at the door."

When Dr. Zydlo got heated up, he did not hesitate to take immediate corrective action. If that involved some hurt feelings, so be it. Zydlo was ever mindful that the paramedics had to perform. When dealing with human lives, failure was not an option. If there were any issues with their performance, attitude, or work ethic, Zydlo cut that off at the ankles. He had no "Plan B". Plan A involved perfection. It did not allow for mistakes or incompetence.

He had trained them up to a standard beyond anything anyone had ever seen. They were not only good, some of them were brilliant. The initial group went into the street and saved lives. They did it in every conceivable condition and in magnificent and brave ways that no one in the medical community could argue with or find fault.

The first men who were really the founding fathers of all paramedics thereafter were a special group. These men had to perform. There was no room for error. If they began screwing up and killing patients because they forgot what they were taught, became nervous---whatever the reason or excuse---their collective performance could absolutely kill the program. They all understood explicitly that what they were embarking on with Zydlo, he would tell them "You guys want to be a wolf? You have to *earn* wolf status. Nobody gives it to you."

The original one hundred and seven paramedics quickly became rock stars. They saved lives and grateful citizens wrote letters to the editor. People quickly took notice. This was a phenomenon not previously seen in medicine.

Palatine, IL. Paramedic Dale Collier

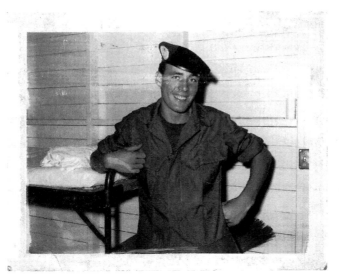

Palatine IL Fire Department paramedic Dale Collier in Vietnam.
Courtesy Dale Collier.

If Dr. Zydlo was Frank Sinatra, then Dale Collier was Elvis. Collier had the full pedigree. War hero, Hollywood good looking, women wanted him, men wanted to be him. Little kids and old ladies adored him. He was treading on legend status.

If Zydlo's number was "92", (the number of children killed in the 1958 Our Lady of the Angels fire) Palatine Fire Department Paramedic Dale Collier's number was "90", as in ninety feet. Collier was the typical Zydlo paramedic. Street smart and brave beyond belief, Collier returned from Vietnam with a chest full of medals and real life experiences of being shot at and hit.

After Vietnam he was working at AT&T and bored out of his mind when he ran into an old family friend who was the Palatine, Illinois Fire Chief. After a very short recruitment pitch from the Chief, Collier decided he wanted to be a fireman and was willing to take an $8,000 pay cut to do so. Though he had a couple of kids and a mortgage, he decided on the spot to join the fire department. This was in spite of a recent fire that had taken the lives of three Palatine firemen, two of whom had been in Zydlo's first paramedic class. But the recent tragic demise of three guys did not affect Colliers' decision in the least. He felt challenged. Man, bring that shit on.

Collier was not in the first class of paramedics, but Zydlo realized early on that Collier was perhaps the most naturally talented paramedic he had ever trained. He had a second sense about the job. He almost never made a mistake. He was a frigging maniac outside of work, but man, send him on any call imaginable and he was textbook perfect. Zydlo quickly had him train other paramedics. He sent him all over the country to teach and to advise television shows on paramedic procedures and practices.

In a 1976 book called *The Paramedics,* author James O. Page[5] recounts an ambulance ride with Collier. The section titled, "The Queen of Palatine" is reprinted below with permission:

THE QUEEN OF PALATINE

It was one of the coldest days in Illinois history. The paramedic ambulance hurtled across icy streets en route to a reported diabetic coma. Arriving at the dismal overgrown bungalow, paramedics Dale Collier, Dave Riddle and Steve Zimmerman bail out of the ambulance with armloads of equipment and bound through the deep snow into the sagging abode.

The interior of the house is a nightmare. Heavy black soot has stained everything, including a frightened dog which races for the door. The kitchen sink is filled with a soot-covered liquid and a filthy cat languishes on the counter, watching the scene with little obvious concern. A defective oil furnace belches smoke into the putrid dwelling. Seated in a chair is Margaret. "Let's get her out of here," Collier commands.

As Margaret is escorted carefully through the snow, she presents a surreal image. Her exposed skin is dark as coal. Her hair is a matted black tangle. She is wrapped in several layers of filthy winter garments. On her feet are a pair of ill-fitting men's shoes. The paramedics don't notice the filth as they clutch her firmly on the short passage to the ambulance.

Inside the warm vehicle, the stench of clothing soaked with body wastes is almost overpowering. But no one seems to notice. Margaret objects briefly as Collier commences to peel off the layers of rags. They are among her few possessions.

Collier is authoritative but sensitive, demanding but comforting. His credentials need not be displayed on his uniform.

Margaret instantly believes in him. She is lowered to the gurney and urged to lay back. The stench of increment regenerates with her movements. A symphony of well-practiced movements begins as the paramedics go to work. Margaret is preoccupied with Collier's questions. "Do you take any medications?" "Are you a diabetic?" "Do you have a headache?" "Have you been nauseous?"

Her answers disclose that she is alert and probably well educated. She hardly notices that Collier has lifted her soiled undershirt and is applying patches. Collier calls for an IV. Riddle has anticipated it. The hospital is contacted. A strip is running and the quick rhythmic squiggle is broken irregularly by PVCs. As Collier tells the lady about the pending IV, he is rechecking heart and breathing sounds, pulling at a grubby stocking to check for swelling ankles. Riddle hits the brittle diabetic vein on the first try. The hospital authorizes transport.

Underway—Zimmerman drives, Collier and Riddle are in perpetual motion. Collier is standing, half-bent over the patient, bracing himself with every bump and turn of the vehicle. Riddle sends another strip. Collier checks breathing sounds, adjusts oxygen flow, replaces a nasal cannula with a mask, and keeps talking. "Are you comfortable, Margaret?" "Do you know who I am?" ("You're a par-a-medic," she responds) "Don't go to sleep now." "Take a deep breath, dear; like this" (demonstrating).

As we pull into the hospital driveway, Margaret vomits. Collier and Riddle grab to get her upright. A pan appears from a cabinet. The odor of vomit has no visible impact on their sensitive concern for this wretched human being. At 9:00 a.m., Margaret was alone, miserable and on the brink of death—a victim of age, poverty, pride, loneliness, the coldest winter in a hundred years, and an oil furnace that had been poisoning her for days.

But at 11:00 a.m. on a January day in 1977, she was the Queen of Palatine, the sole object of concern and skill of three young paramedics.

Seventy-three years of life and some tough breaks could put most of us in a similar situation of misery and despair.

Let's hope we will have the security of emergency medical services that really care, that will treat without concern for ability to pay, that won't judge a patient by appearances or odors, that will respond without question, delay or red tape.

Page was a prolific writer and promoter of the paramedic movement. He, perhaps above anyone else in those early days, was responsible for spreading the gospel. In the article featuring Collier, he captures the spirit and professional competence of a paramedic at the top of his game. The heroic stuff happened every 200 runs or so. "The Queen of Palatine" stuff happened every day. This is what endeared the paramedics to the community. They were consistent, professional, and competent. They were seldom rattled. They never panicked and always showed up.

Collier, a decorated real life Vietnam War hero, had certainly seen his share of blood and gore in just about every conceivable manner. In the case that resulted in the "90" designation, he rolled up on a guy who had fallen off a water tower from a height of ninety feet and landed on the concrete pad surrounding the water tower base. This was a new one for Collier. The first thought that ran through his mind was "No fucking way this guy is alive."

Saving the Tower Rat

Robert Lee Turner, a 27-year-old native of Henderson, Kentucky, worked for Service Enterprise, out of Evansville, Indiana. On this day, November 26, 1982, he was in Palatine, Illinois, cutting down an old water tower tank that would be replaced by a larger water tank. It was cold, snowy, and foggy---a classic, miserable Chicago hawk blowing day. Depending upon who you talk to, he was either 105 feet or 80 feet in the air, using a cutting torch. He made one cut too many, was pulled off and fell a hundred feet or so to the ground,

As his terrified co-worker, Michael Oldhan, looked on, Turner hit a concrete pad below the tower like a ripe watermelon. He landed on his hands and knees and looked very dead. Four months prior, Scott Shedler of Buffalo Grove, Illinois had been climbing the same tower and fell from thirty-five feet. He died from his injuries. Turner had just fallen almost three times that distance

When Dale Collier and his partner, Ed Kemper, arrived and assessed the damage, the only thing Collier, a veteran of multiple tours of duty in Vietnam and had witnessed some horrific combat, could think of was this guy "feels like a bag of doorknobs." Every major bone in his body was broken. He appeared to be bleeding out of every orifice---and, holy shit, he was breathing. Collier went to work on the victim. He plugged holes and assessed the damage.

A terrified 19-year-old kid up on top of the tower gave Ed Kemper a very different problem. The kid was freaked out, not moving or responding to either Kemper or Collier. The longest ladder truck they had could only reach 70 feet, a huge issue since the kid was about a hundred feet off the ground. Even the Arlington Heights ladder truck couldn't reach high enough. Kemper decided to go get him before they had two victims on the concrete.

Short of bringing in a helicopter, Kemper knew the only way up was to use the construction crane that had been used to assist to dismantle the water tower. It is, or at least on this day seems to be, the world's largest and most dangerous erector set. Except this isn't a child's toy. This is a real, fifty-ton behemoth steel monster, all angles and cold, hard American made steel made for heavy duty construction work involving tonnage. When the mechanical engineers designed and built this monster, they did not take into consideration that men would climb on it for any reason.

Kemper and Jensen were not gymnasts or Olympic athletes. They had never, prior to this moment, considered climbing up the side of one of these beasts. It's cold, really cold. It's windy and snowing. The metal is freezing. If you touch it with your bare hand, you'll leave a few layers of skin behind. No handles or steps to use. Every step is fraught with danger. None of the bars are level and they're all welded at severe angles. The thing looks like a torture chamber of monkey bars for adults.

The crane had more than enough length, so Kemper and Emil Jensen, an off-duty firefighter who lived nearby, began the long, laborious, and dangerous climb to retrieve Michael Oldhan.

He had one way up. The crane was still in place. As soon as he started to climb, Kemper realized that his safety line would be too short. Crawling up a crane boom was not easy. All the materials were steel. There were no hand or foot holds.

None of that matters when you have a potential second victim on top of a tower, so Kemper moved up those iron cross beams like a toddler on a sugar high. When he finally got to the top and looked down, he realized for real that from this height there was the potential to kill all of them. Kemper was in great shape, but between the climb and the mental aspect of this incident, he was quickly gassed and operating on pure adrenaline.

He found Oldhan in shock, freezing, not responding, and curled, with a death grip, around the remaining guardrail on top the tower. Kemper had to figure out how to get him down without killing all three of them. There was no easy way. They would have to climb back down the same dangerous way they went up.

Kemper knew it was all bad. There was zero room for error. He had no idea how to get himself and the kid down the side of a construction crane. Who said this job was fun? Clearly whoever said it was not standing ninety-something feet in the air with no plan as to how to get down while basically carrying a fully grown man who, by the looks of him, had not missed many meals lately.

Kemper and Jensen finally got a harness and safety lines on Oldhan who was wrapped around the guardrail like it was his prom date. They pried him off and the three of them duck-walked down the crane without any further drama, although this is an extremely inadequate description of the danger and heroics of this little exercise.

No human in his right mind would think about climbing up and down this thing in any conditions. Today, fire departments of most any size have highly-trained specialists who manage these problems. There is no chance that a couple of paramedics, untrained on high climbing would jump on this crane to attempt any kind of rescue. But forty years ago the options were---well, there were no other options. Consequently, Kemper and Jensen performed their little miracle in the sky with close to zero fanfare, save a couple of newspaper articles.

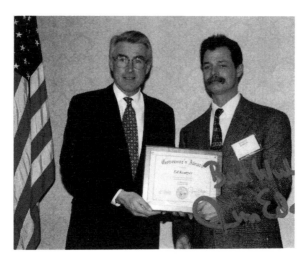

IL Governor Jim Edgar presenting Palatine Paramedic Ed Kemper the Medal of Honor. Courtesy Ed Kemper.

Michael Oldhan has never been interviewed, but he has told close friends he will never speak of this incident again.

Robert Lee Turner, tougher than old, rusty sheet metal and with the scars to prove it, recalls that when he came to there were a half dozen doctors standing over his hospital bed. Everything was more than a little murky. One old guy was talking and all Robert could remember was that he was told he would never walk again. Then, they started with a laundry list of his injuries. The highlights are as follows:

1. Crushed pelvis
2. All his ribs were fractured
3. Broken jaw
4. Severe concussion
5. Two broken arms
6. Left elbow was shattered
7. Lung punctured
8. Liver lacerated into two pieces
9. Stomach lacerated
10. Torn Rotator cuffs
11. Multiple fractures of both legs
12. Hip broken
13. More stitches than he could count. Literally hundreds of them
14. From the waist down, full cast

Now an active, over-the-road truck driver, Robert Lee Turner fully recovered and has led a productive life as a father and grandfather. He is convinced that he would not have survived the fall had Dale Collier not been on his "A" game. The subsequent, excellent surgeons who put him back together did a right fair job, as well.

Dale Collier, who was also a Captain at the time, was later credited with dozens of saves over the years, but he could not recall hearing or knowing about an accident victim who fell from that distance and even came close to surviving. The actions of Collier, Kemper and Jensen no doubt contributed to this incident not turning into an even greater disaster.

Ed Kemper eventually retired due to Kemper medical issues, but even though retired, it was not the end of his heroics. On October 25, 1995, Ed Kemper, as was his custom, was up and out of the house to go work out. He was then 40 years old and still in incredible physical condition. At this writing, he is 60 years old and in better physical condition then most professional athletes. His dedication to "Cross Fit"[6] has served him well to this day.

October 25, 1995
Fox River Grove Tragedy

Kemper had just picked up his coffee at a White Hen store, and was pumping gas into his truck, when he heard a commuter train whistle screaming non-stop. He was in Fox River Grove, Illinois, a sleepy little suburb of Chicago, where he had watched trains come down those tracks most of his adult life. He knew what a regular train whistle sounded like and knew instantly what he was hearing was anything but normal.

As he looked up, his heart jumped right out of his chest because sitting on the railroad tracks, and clearly not moving, was a full-sized school bus packed with kids. Kemper did what he always did. He set out for the school bus on a dead run because he knew that in seconds a disaster would happen.

Kemper ran across a four-lane highway and watched as 500 tons of steel, in the form of a packed Chicago area commuter train, whipped down at 70mph headed right for the parked, school bus sitting right in the center of its gunsights.

The bus sat immobile on the tracks like a big fat yellow target and Kemper screamed at it to get off the tracks. Too late. That commuter train hit that bus and just demolished it. Unfortunately, there were 35 teenagers and a substitute bus driver on the bus. Kemper watched the train hit that bus and twenty years later he is positive of one thing. He never, not once in decades of service had ever seen anything like this. The train hit the bus with such energy the entire bus separated its chassis.

Kemper didn't hesitate. He was on that demolished bus seconds after the train hit it. For the next 40 minutes, Kemper triaged and brought some order to the worst train/school bus accident in the history of the United States. Kemper hit that bus in full stride. He was on it for about three seconds before he realized that it would be a miracle if anyone survived the devastation that appeared before him.

Immediately, he got the walking wounded out of the way. The most serious damage was in the rear. A lot of the kids saw the train coming and started running towards the front before the accident occurred. They were the lucky ones because their injuries were the least life threatening. Kemper quickly got them off the bus and told them all to stay put. He then had the additional problem of civilians attempting to pull victims off the bus.

He began to scream at people to not touch the victims as the kids were coming out of the shock of being hit by a train. The pain, shock, and agony kicked into high gear. He had a million tasks to accomplish with the sum total of an ink pen and a pocketknife in his pocket. That was it----the biggest disaster to ever hit a small community and Kemper has to make do with no equipment and no help.

Kemper would later reflect on this and think that on the hundreds and hundreds of calls he had responded to throughout the years, he always had a big advantage. He would be in the firehouse and the call would come in. He and his partners would jump in the ambulance and immediately start talking over a plan of action, what equipment they would need, as well as other backup or assistance. This always mentally prepared him for what he was rolling up on. It was the calm before the storm that always afforded him an edge. Not today. On this day, the world's biggest shit storm had just fallen down on top of him. Zero time and zero equipment. For all practical purposes, he was standing there in his underwear.

In the rear of the bus where the carnage was at its worst, Kemper tried to identify the dead and those out of reach who needed help the quickest. Finally, an off duty Mt. Prospect fireman, Brendon Keedy, arrived. Keedy had even less equipment then Kemper, but he was at least another professional who was immensely helpful.

Finally, after about forty minutes, Kemper had triaged the kids. He and Keedy had the victims on boards and handed them off to local fire personnel to get them to various area hospitals. The entire time that Kemper and Keedy were in that bus no one else entered and helped. Everyone stood outside of the bus letting Kemper run the entire scene. Eventually, all of the surviving victims got off the bus. As Kemper was getting off the bus, covered in blood from head to toe, one of the kids he had told to get off the bus was standing right where he was told to be.

His name was Jason Kedrok and he had held the students who were the walking wounded together. Kedrok would later become a fireman himself and twenty years to the date of this tragedy was now working in Arlington Heights, Illinois where he works for, and with, many of Ed Kemper's old contemporaries and friends. Ed and Jason have remained close through the years.

In the aftermath of this disaster, Kemper was awarded the state's highest Medal of Honor award and an armful of others, as well. Out of the 35 children on that bus, seven did not make it, but for Ed Kemper's actions that day, that number could have been much higher, proving Zydlo's genius once again.

Steve Johnson, Paramedic, EMS Director, Schaumburg Fire Department

Steve Johnson has been a paramedic since he was about 19 when he lied about his age and was able to sneak into Zydlo's training group.

Zydlo caught him, and after some time thinking about it, he decided to let Johnson stay. Zydlo always had a soft spot for the rascals.

Johnson eventually became one of the first paramedics in the Chicago Fire Department. After four years of working the west side of Chicago, he went to the Schaumburg Fire Department in Schaumburg, Illinois. Today, he is the EMS coordinator in a city of 74,000. He supervises 88 full time paramedics who make 6,600 ambulance runs a year in their city. In 1973, when Johnson trained in the third class taught by Zydlo, he never dreamed he would be in the position he has currently held for nine years. He almost did not reach this position because when he was 52 years old and working out in the firehouse on the treadmill, he suffered a massive heart attack. To add insult to injury, he cracked his head open in the fall and received a skull fracture.

Luckily for him, his paramedics were able to shock him, perform CPR, and bring him back to life. This would be a reoccurring theme throughout the history of these paramedics because the paramedics even saved Dr. Zydlo when he had a heart attack at home.

On Good Friday in 1983, Johnson received a call about a traffic accident involving a Kinder Care bus. There was no report of any injuries. When he and his partner arrived at the accident scene, it was yet another vision from hell. Scattered and laying in the street were at least a dozen small children. Civilian, non-emergency vehicles and a large crowd were making the scene even more chaotic.

The kids would not make their appointment to visit the Easter Bunny. One child was dead, a woman driving a Cadillac, who was hit head on by the Kinder Care bus, was dead. A few kids were not breathing and others had dozens of serious injuries. What started out as a simple traffic accident was, in reality, another disaster involving young children.

Whenever Stan Zydlo reflected back on this tragedy, he always looked upon it with pride. He credited Johnson's cool head under fire with making sure this accident did not turn out much worse than it did. There were a lot of kids in critical condition and Zydlo felt that Johnson was primarily responsible for saving many of them.

Johnson deflects the praise simply saying, "It was a team effort and I just did my job."

Zydlo, however, remembered Johnson's heroics on that Good Friday very differently. Nevertheless, no matter whose memory is more correct, there is this. Johnson, like all of his brethren who have gone above and beyond the call of duty, has saved thousands of lives in his long and storied career.

They all do it to the detriment of their health, their families, and their own well-being. They do it in the snow, the rain, and heat. They do it under every conceivable adverse condition. They never take a day off. They are there whenever they are needed, and they do it better and more consistently then any other similar type agency anyone can think of.

Paramedic William Dressel, Arlington Heights, IL FD, (Retired)

And show up they did. Take, for example, Bill Dressel, who was in the first paramedic class. He showed up rain or shine for the next forty years without fail. He would still be working, but he reached the mandatory retirement age and the Arlington Heights paramedic had to hang it up. Dressel started with AHFD in 1968. In those pre-paramedic days, Dressel recalls the simpler times.

"It was real easy when we had a bad accident, we just called the funeral home and told them where to go."

That soon changed. He jumped head over heels into the paramedic program. He embraced it from the beginning and never looked back. To look at Dressel today, one would never guess that he's eligible for the early bird special at Denny's because he looks fifteen years younger than his real age.

Many of the paramedics that started in '72 burned out, got promoted, or just went on to finish their career doing something different then working the Ambo. Not Bill Dressel. Year in and year out, Bill passed the recertification test. From 1972 through 2009, Dressel rode that Ambo. That is just shy of 41 years. He never considered doing anything else. The only reason he is not bouncing around the streets today is mandatory retirement rules. His longevity and expertise as a paramedic was second to no one.

Dressel lives in a neat as a pin, oversized ranch home in a near west suburb of Chicago. The house is so pristine and neat you could eat off the floor. He restores old hot rods and works out every day without fail. He is in great shape and he looks it. It is surprising that someone hasn't made a reality show about him yet, but Dressel, like so many of his colleagues, is uninterested. That is not him and never will be.

It may just be his base personality, or it may be the fact that he has been witness to more human misery then ten people see in a lifetime. As one can imagine, Dressel worked everything from plane crashes and catastrophic accidents to split lips and migraines. His institutional knowledge of the job was encyclopedic. When he left the AHFD, that information and experience could never be replaced.

In forty plus years, Bill had dozens of saves. He minimizes his role in these things as most of the men and woman do. His colleagues do not minimize his contributions. Bill's bosses loved him because he always showed up, gave 110%, never bitched, and was friend, mentor, and team player to his last day. His peers and co-workers describe him as "Dedicated, hardworking, conscientious, whip smart," and say that "He always acted in the best interests of his patients."

Bill would only comment on one save and predictably it was a heart attack. He is an expert in CPR. He so good, so competent, he teaches it to medical doctors and dentists. Heart attacks are definitely in his wheelhouse. No doubt about that and it's a good thing because one of Bill's greatest saves involved a heart attack victim.

It's always starts out simply. A voice comes over the speaker in the firehouse. "Man having chest pains." The ambulance rolls and any paramedic in the country knows how to play this. It is almost never complicated. This is why they get the big bucks. Slap some aspirin in the patient, give oxygen, start an IV, slap a blood pressure cup on, and off you go to help pay for the cardiologist's Porsche.

Not this time. This time the dude was coding and it was all going to hell on an express train. He's in his forties, a little overweight, but definitely not in visual heart attack territory. It doesn't matter. Chubby Guy is going down fast and when the troops blasted through that front door, none of them would have given any odds on Chubby guy wolfing down another cheeseburger this time tomorrow.

It was Chubby Guy's good Karma day because running the show was Bill Dressel who knew this would, in the old days, have been a funeral home call. That was the old days. It's a new day and the master is in the house. In the time it took Dressel to cross the room and take a look at Chubby Guy, he already knew he was in deep. Chubby Guy was not conscious but had a faint pulse.

Dressel started CPR and the guy came back for a moment. He coded again. Bam! Once again Dressel dragged him back from the brink of eating an unlimited supply of Snicker bars in Heaven. Dressel and the boys got him to the hospital and Chubby Guy survived in time to hit the midnight buffet at Steak & Shake.

Dressel readily recalls the bad ones---and to call them bad is perhaps an understatement. The worst call he was ever involved in was a house fire around Christmas that was started by an errant smoker in the home. When the smoke cleared three generations of family members were dead. None of the seven victims in the house had a chance. The smoke and toxic fumes got all of them. Some were very young children. Those are the cases that you see in your dreams for years to come. It never gets easy.

Another call was one of the first the fire department responded to after becoming part of EMS. It was shortly after the creation of the program. It may have been one of the very first calls. It was in the middle of the night and within minutes two calls came in from opposite ends of town. Ambulances 515 and 516 rolled and each victim was having a heart attack. This is very unusual in a city of this size. On this night, neither victim was revived.

They lost them both and the responding paramedics were crushed. It was an unusual occurrence. They had had some great successes early and this one hurt bad. Although it was the early days of the program, they all knew they were good. The saves were coming fast and furious from all over Zydlo's network and expectations of not losing anyone were becoming unrealistic. The first rule in emergency medicine is simple, "Not everyone lives". You run off a string of victories and the tendency is to start believing you will not lose one. It's all good until your old nemesis, death, walks up and smacks you in the face a few times.

As Dr. Zydlo always advised, "Don't get too high with the highs and don't get too low with the lows." It was, as usual, sage advice.

Lieutenant Berny Goss, Elk Grove, IL Fire Department, (Retired)

Most of the paramedics had military backgrounds. They were used to being placed in high stress situations. Zydlo's act was different in that what he taught was not so much physical. The job itself involved a lot of physical activity, but it was manageable, especially if you were in decent shape. No, this job required some brains and a lot of common sense. You had to have both. The firemen generally had a ton of common sense, but not many were known as cerebral, deep thinkers.

In Berny Goss's case, he had brains and a lot of them. He did not come from the military. He came from CPS---Chicago Public Schools. Bernie was a teacher there when he decided that hustling the little darlings in and out of math class all day was not very much fun. He knew there had to be something out there that was a little more challenging then teaching high school, so he did what all good Irish boys who grew up on Chicago's south side Bridgeport neighborhood did. He found himself a public service job in the fast growing suburban Elk Grove Village that borders O'Hare airport on its northwest side of Chicago. There is a lot of manufacturing and industry in Elk Grove Village and the fire department stays busy.

Berny was hired almost immediately after taking the test for the fire department. His timing was near perfect. It was a good job, but Berny was bored. There were moments of excitement, but they were few and far between. After about two years on the job, Berny heard about the paramedic program and was raring to go. However, he had a very pregnant wife at home and he missed the inaugural class. He enrolled in the second Zydlo paramedic class while concurrently attending EMT school at Loyola.

Berny was unusual because unlike the vast majority of his colleagues, he had a four-year degree. Today, this is far from unusual. Back when Berny got on the job, it was as rare as Mickey Mantle playing sober. Berny though, bright guy that he was, found his calling. Not many people knew how this would play out, but Berny found Zydlo to be unlike any medical doctor he would meet in the next several decades of working around emergency rooms and hospitals. He thought that Zydlo was brilliant. He was clearly a superior teacher to any instructor or teacher Berny had ever had. "He was also pretty damn scary," Bernie said, chuckling, over forty years later. "Stan taught like he practiced medicine. He was intense and laser beam focused in everything he did. He also expected you to get it quick and get it right. If you didn't…and I'm not kidding…he looked like he would beat the shit out of you right there."

Zydlo was not for the faint-hearted or timid.

Berny soaked this stuff up. He hit full stride early and was one of Zydlo's early stars. Rock steady and always present in the moment, Berny had a very supportive chief. He loved the work. He was the typical "Zydlo trained medic". Steady and smart, he always had the ability to do the right thing at the right time. He seldom made a mistake and, like many of those early paramedics, it was because of his very steady hands that the paramedic program flourished in this country.

For his part, Zydlo usually knew very early on in the course who would wind up being a star. He was certain of Goss and was right, as usual.

Goss had a thirty-year career full of great saves. Like many of the other early paramedics, Goss was as steady at home as he was on the job. He and his wife Kathleen have been married for over fifty years. They have lived in the same house for over fifty years and they raised four children who also turned out to be fairly steady. Their son is one of the youngest deputy chiefs of police in the nation at a large, very busy Chicago suburban department. Two of their daughters are nurses and the last daughter is a schoolteacher who Berny is most proud of because, as he said, "She figured out how to work even less days then I did."

Zydlo was an intimidating figure, but he was fair. He barked and yelled at everyone. There were no exceptions. But as you saw it all coming together, you started to understand the gravity of what you would be doing and why he (Zydlo) was such a hot wire. Berny thought about this whole

"*Zydlo trained medic*" stuff and he thought that what it really meant was that Stan made you feel "courageous". Zydlo made you feel competent and courageous enough to make split second life and death decisions. He also stressed how critical it was to be always prepared for any emergency. Berny thought that this was perhaps Zydlo's greatest gift to his paramedics.

Goss was also a little unusual in that he worked full time at the fire department while attending EMT and paramedic school simultaneously. Reflecting back, Goss has one real distinct memory about those days. As he was in both the EMT and paramedic programs at the same time, he was in a very unique position. He heard two very different ways of teaching being thrown at him and they were as about as different as it can get, but it was also very useful.

On more than one occasion in the EMT class he would break out something Zydlo had taught him in the previous night's paramedic course. The younger guys would look at him in amazement and say, "Hey, are you a doctor or something?" Goss would just say "No guys. I'm just a *Zydlo trained paramedic*". Goss knew at moments like this he was really learning stuff that was not on the Boy Scout merit badge test for first aid.

As a paramedic you go through this very intense and often very difficult training and you start to gain some real confidence. It seems to come all together at once, but there is one little detail left and, as several paramedics put it, "You ain't saved one patient and man you just aren't sure you are going to perform like you were trained."

Berny Goss was no exception to this rule. The fact that this paramedic thing was brand new and no one had any idea how it would play out qualified this as a very valid feeling. That all changed fairly quickly. Berny's first call as a paramedic was to a familiar address. The fire department had been to this home numerous times because a young girl, who was a juvenile (brittle) diabetic, lived there. It was the same routine every time. Race there, grab the kid and haul ass to the hospital so the ER people could save her.

Now it was different, very different, because they had trained for this. The treatment protocol was simple. Get some glucose and an IV into the patient and they should be ok. Great theory, but if you have never done it, it is still a theory. So they get the call and race out. Racing out there is Goss, another paramedic and three engine guys and the parents are right there along with the victim. The victim is out. This is very serious and the stakes are very high.

One, it's a young girl, (kids are not supposed to be this sick or die). Two, this is happening more frequently, thus raising the chances that this kid is running out of lucky breaks. Brain damage is a distinct possibility, as is death. Berny gets the IV started, pumps some glucose into the kid and Bam! She comes right to and is right as rain. The parents cry tears of joy and relief. The EMS personnel are also close to crying. Damn, if it didn't work just like they were taught. At that moment, they all understood. It hit them hard. Everyone in that small bungalow knew without a doubt that a miracle had just happened right in front of all of them in living color.

This was not training. It was not a story they were reading about in Readers Digest. This was exactly how the plan was supposed to work. They may not quite claim this as saving a life, but tell that young girl's parents that this was not lifesaving stuff. For those brand new paramedics, this type of call would become so routine, so predictable, it would qualify as easy. A year from then their collective pulse rates wouldn't rise, even slightly, on a call like this.

The calls were as varied as the human condition. They learned this on the run and it and they were becoming so good that the general public, as well as the medical establishment, were figuring out just how invaluable the paramedics were becoming. The paramedics and Zydlo never got comfortable. They were learning hard lessons every day and they knew that every call was different.

As Berny explains, "We found out you could not do this alone. The engine guys, the rescue squad rolled with us on every call. We were figuring this out together and that was what really cranked up our skill level and confidence. It was that collective institutional knowledge that we gained and always passed on to the younger guys and girls who were coming up."

Zydlo had such a high opinion of Berny he sent him out to California, along with Dale Collier, to work with the paramedics operating in Los Angeles County.

The LA guys ran a similar skill set as Zydlo's guys with one difference---*they didn't transport patients.* They showed up at the scene and did what they could. Then a private ambulance company would transport the patient to the hospital. They were not operating in a mobile intensive care unit or ambulance. They would treat at the scene and release, ending their participation. Zydlo's guys treated right up to the handoff at the emergency room.

Berny and Collier were also guests of the hit TV show *Emergency,* a television series that combined the medical drama and action-adventure genres. It debuted on NBC on January 15, 1972. The series starred Randolph Mantooth and Kevin Tighe as two specially trained firefighters, who formed Squad 51, part of the then innovative field of paramedics authorized to provide initial emergency medical care to victims of accidents, fires, and other incidents in the field.[7]

The television show raised the profile of paramedics to such a degree that politicos started (reluctantly) getting serious about prehospital care and especially the funding issues faced with the addition of these skilled personnel.

Collier and Goss were invited to the set, where the stars of the show treated them like stars. Collier was not impressed. He could not believe that Hollywood let him go back home without offering him a TV show.

Berny Goss, like most every other suburban paramedic, bristles when asked if Chicago, Boston, New York, or any large fire department paramedics, are better than their suburban counterparts because they often (depending on the assigned firehouse) deal with a much larger volume of calls. Based on that criteria, the answer is, "No." The suburban paramedics just may have a valid point because the fact is anything that has ever happened in a large city has also happened in smaller towns.

When Berny Goss started his shift on May 25, 1979, American Airlines Flight 191 was a regularly scheduled passenger flight operated by American Airlines from O'Hare International Airport in Chicago to Los Angeles International Airport. The McDonnell Douglas DC10 crashed moments after takeoff from Chicago. All 258 passengers and 13 crew on board were killed, along with two people on the ground. It was the deadliest aviation accident in the United States.[8]

The first ambulance on the scene belonged to Berny Goss. He had a relatively young paramedic with him who would later become chief of the department. When they arrived at the scene, the entire crash site was covered with dead passengers and multiple fires. To further complicate matters, the plane just had departed with a full tank of gas. Thousands and thousands of gallons of jet fuel were almost guaranteed to explode, causing even further damage and loss of life. Goss and his partner were right in the middle of this.

While Goss was contemplating their next move, his younger partner asked him, "What are we going to do?" Berny looked around at the horribly dismembered and burned beyond recognition laying over a several hundred-yard area and replied, "Nothing. They are all dead."

He was right because, as explained later by other firemen who came to the scene, "We didn't see one body intact, just trunks, hands, arms, heads, and parts of legs. And we can't tell whether they were male or female, or whether they were adult or child, because they were all charred."

A First Responder on the scene stated, "It was too hot to touch anybody and I really couldn't tell if they were men or women."[9]

The immediate problem was the dozens of raging fires that were getting closer by the second to the unburned fuel. As Goss looked over towards the airport, through the high security chain link fence, there came a big beautiful Chicago fire truck, and it was flying. Now Goss knew very little about the Chicago Fire Department operation at the airport, but he knew they were forbidden to leave airport property for a variety of serious reasons. There were no exceptions to this rule.

Goss and his partner were way off the property line of the airport so for the life of himself he could not begin to guess why the oversized fire truck was still coming at them. Clearly, it had no equipment that could reach them. "What the hell were these guys doing? The big red beast was cooking and picking up momentum the closer it got. It was also running out of runway and it was still picking up speed as it hit the grass that surrounded the airfield doing fifty or sixty miles per hour. It kept right on charging toward the crash site and now all that stood between Goss and the truck was that big ass ten-foot security fence that encircled the entire airport property. It hit the fence and flattened it, then rolled into that crash site like an avenging angel. Rules and regs be damned, they were way off the property and no doubt someone was going to get their ass fried over this one. Nevertheless, it did not matter because as we have read, the brotherhood, the oath, and the code that these men and women make towards each other trumps all rules that most mortals would follow.

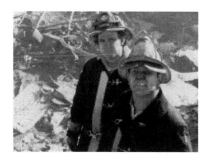

Elk Grove Villiage Paramedic Berny Goss (R), and Paramedic Doug Goostree
on scene at Flight 191 crash on May 25, 1979.

They hit those fires with the chemical compound designed to fight these extremely dangerous fires and extinguished it in short order. To put it mildly, Goss and his partner were happy that the CFD guys did not stand on formalities. It was a bad day for the victims and their family members, but for Goss it just reinforced what he knew then and continuing on through the day he retired. He would miss the clowns, but he would happily leave the circus behind.

Lieutenant Francis O'Shea, Schaumburg IL Fire Department, (Active)

No one keeps these records, but when you are perhaps the second youngest person (after his brother Pat) to have ever attended the paramedic class, the youngest person to ever work as a paramedic in a fire department and, finally, having the longest continuing employment (44 years as a fireman/paramedic), you can absolutely believe that you will be a part of the historical record that eventually names names.

Schaumburg Fire Department Lt. Francis J. O'Shea Jr., is part of a lineage of fire department royalty. On his own, Fran O'Shea is one of the best known and highly respected firefighters to ever strap on bunker or turnout gear. He would cringe and deny all of these things because that is just the kind of guy he is. Old school all the way, he is the ultimate standard bearer for the Brotherhood. Duty, honor, and protecting the brotherhood are not just words tossed about at happy hour and fireman funerals. They are his way of life. It is concrete stamped into his DNA.

Anyone looking at O'Shea's personnel file would, in all likelihood, come to the same conclusion and yet a closer look could give pause because it is entirely possible that Lt. Francis O'Shea may not even be the best fireman/paramedic in his own family. That sort of thing happens when you are part of five generations of firemen with a family history going back to June 1, 1890.

Fran's great grandfather, George F. "Bull" Kelly, strapped on some Chicago Fire Department gear, raised his right hand, and started the life driving a horse pulled fire equipment laden wagon throughout the streets of Chicago. His salary for these duties was approximately $1,300.00 a year.

Chicago firefighters labored under the "continuous duty system" which required them to live at their fire stations day and night with only three breaks for meals. With luck, a fireman would receive a day off from this routine once or twice a month and, depending upon the disposition of his fire chief, vacation breaks.[10] One hundred and twenty-six years later, the Kelly/O'Shea clan is still at it.

In the grand and long history of the Irish and the CFD, a hardworking/hard-charging fireman was known to occasionally partake in a glass of beer or a spirit or two. "Bull" Kelly was alleged to have participated in these activities while on duty. "Bull's" personnel file makes note of some events.

He was not known to endear himself to management. In spite of getting regular promotions on an almost annual basis, he also managed to piss off the bosses fairly regularly. For example, on May 3, 1894, Bull was cited (found guilty of) intoxication and verbal abuse. It is suspected that he may have done a bit more then "verbally abuse" someone because on May 26, 1894, Bull was fired from the CFD.

After an eleven-month vacation, Bull reinstated to the CFD. Apparently all was forgiven because one year later he was promoted again. Bull may have jumped in a twelve-step program because for the next several years he managed to avoid any alleged, or real, bad behavior. In fact, on December 30, 1903, Bull Kelly and his colleagues responded to a fire at the old Iroquois Theater located at 79-81 Randolph Street at 3:32 p.m. Bull received a CFD commendation for rescuing a disabled lady from an upper floor balcony.

On December 22, 1910, he was involved in fighting a fire at the Chicago Stockyards where twenty-one of his brothers were killed while attempting to put out a raging fire. In 1913, Bull Kelly retired from the CFD after twenty-three years of service. The die was cast and the Kelly/O'Shea clan's future was committed to the brotherhood.

Lt. Leo S. Kelly, Chicago, Illinois Fire Department

"Bull" Kelly apparently found time in between those month-long shifts to sire some little Bulls. On December 13, 1929, Bull's son, Leo S. Kelly, entered the CFD as a candidate fireman. He was 26. It was bad timing because less than a month later Leo was laid off due to the October 1929 stock market crash that put the entire country into a financial tailspin. Nevertheless, the City scraped up enough dough to reinstate Leo three days later. By 1933, Leo Kelly had received three promotions within thirty months.

However, on July 31, 1934, Leo's bloodline caught up with him when he lost two days' pay for violation of department rules. The record is unclear as to what those violations were, but family rumor suggests Leo (son of "Bull") smacked some boss in the face when the boss got a little rude.

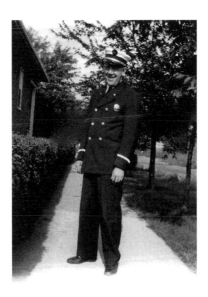

CFD Lt. Leo "Fripo" Kelly grandfather of Fran O'Shea circa 1937. Courtesy O'Shea family.

Apparently Leo did not tolerate bad manners. Then again on January 1, 1937, Leo was forced to donate ten days pay for yet another nitpicky rule violation. There may have been a bit more than a smack in the face on that occasion. Leo, aka "Firpo", got his nickname from the professional prizefighter who knocked World Heavy Weight Champion Jack Dempsey right out of the ring around 1926.

Leo eventually managed to keep his hands busy doing other things because on November 15, 1938 he was awarded the Lambert Tree Medal, CFD's highest award for bravery, after he rescued an invalid, bedridden woman from a second floor bedroom at 1440 N. Milwaukee Ave.

The Lambert Tree Medal is named after a U.S. Ambassador, Jurist, and Patron of the Arts. Judge Lambert Tree was a Chicago Circuit Court judge who achieved fame by presiding over the indictment, trial, and conviction of corrupt city council members. He lost the 1882 U.S. Senate race by one vote, but in 1885 accepted an appointment from President

Grover Cleveland as minister to Belgium. Lambert Tree and Chicago Mayor Carter H. Harrison put up the funding for civilian awards given annually to an individual member of the police and fire departments who demonstrate outstanding bravery in the line of duty. Currently, the medal presentations are rotated from year to year, so neither award is perceived as better than the other. The awards are given out during Fire Prevention Week in October each year for the preceding twelve months. These awards have been presented annually (with the exception of the years 1890-1896) since March 4, 1887.[11]

You might be a hot shit hero, but the CFD and the suits that run it apparently are not impressed with true heroism. On June 11, 1949, CFD finally promoted Leo Kelly to lieutenant and assigned him to the 1st Division CFD Headquarters. It took fifteen years, but Leo finally got his white shirt.

You can take the blue shirt out of the squad, but you can't put a white shirt on him and expect him to become a company man because on August 31, 1949, Lt. Kelly was asked to donate another eight days of pay for expressing himself a little too physically for the boss's taste. Getting promoted to lieutenant must have been a pretty nice bump in pay because again on January 31, 1952, Lt. Kelly gracefully took another five days of work off to consider his on duty activities that for some reason kept causing him to take these unpaid mini vacations. "Firpo" was making "Bull" look like a company man.

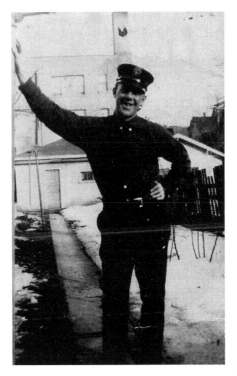

CFD Firefighter Leo Kelly great grandfather of Fran O'Shea circa 1930, Courtesy O'Shea family.

Now either Leo took the cure or those pains in his ass retired, because it was all blue skies and clear sailing. Leo's wife no doubt breathed a sigh of relief because the family rainy day fund suffered no more deductions. In fact, on May 23, 1952, Leo was once again cited for bravery when he rescued a person from the third floor of a burning building at 2124 S. LaSalle St in Chicago at 3:12 am.

On November 15 1952, Lt. Kelly was honored by Mayor Martin Kennelly (who preceded Mayor Richard J. Daley) for heroism and given one of the largest cash prizes in the history of the city. The cash prize was $200 and, considering what a shifty alderman could rake in on a good weekend of graft and corruption, it was insignificant. Then again, Leo was about saving lives, not getting rich. On July 22, 1953, Lieutenant Leo Kelly of Engine 118, son of Bull Kelly, father-in-law of Francis O'Shea, pulled the plug and retired after twenty-three and a half years of heroic service.

Francis O'Shea, Sr., Assistant Chief, Hoffman Estates, Illinois Fire Department

After sixty-three years of service the Kelly/O'Shea clan was just warming up. Francis O'Shea Sr. was a hard working carpenter by trade and profession. In his heart though, at the center of his very soul, he was a fire-fighting son of a bitch.

He was also a WWII vet and a combat medic who fought his way across Europe killing Nazis and saving other combat solders. Because he had a huge family and he had to make a living to support that ever expanding brood, he plied his trade as a master carpenter by day. By night, weekends, holidays and any other free time, he was a volunteer fireman with the Hoffman Estates Fire Department. He married into the Kelly family and he, too, had that firebug glowing inside of his soul.

Many of you reading this know that volunteer firemen/paramedics and women are just as valuable and heroic as their full-time paid colleagues. They drill, they train and they respond just as hard and quickly as the pros. They just do it for free or very low pay. They are the backbone of the fire service in rural areas and smaller towns and they often do it for decades.

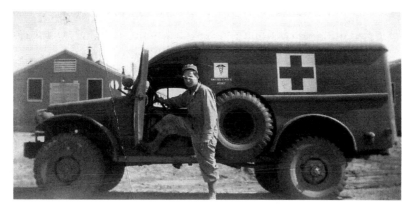

Francis O'Shea Sr., in England during WWII. Coutesy O'Shea family

Make no mistake about their roles. They are as dedicated and competent as humanly possible and while they may get a bad rap in some circles they are as true to the brotherhood as they can be. Throughout the years they have given their lives to the brotherhood and their contributions should never be underestimated.

In 1957, Francis and his wife Lauretta (nee Kelly) moved to the Chicago suburb of Hoffman Estates, located slightly northwest of Chicago. Today, it has approximately 51,000 residents. Its fire department has four separate stations and 96 sworn personnel. When the O'Shea family moved there on Easter Day 1957, the fire department was an all-volunteer operation. Francis Jr. was the oldest child at six years old. It was not an easy transition for Francis Jr. As he explained many years later, "Growing up with the name Francis was not easy. You had two choices with that name. You could run or you could fight and I was not very fast."

For Francis Sr, the name was not an issue because, like the Kelly clan he married into, the O'Sheas were not exactly pacifists. He eventually became a charter member fireman in the history of the village.

Francis Sr. served on the Hoffman Estates FD from 1957 through twenty-three years until they disbanded the volunteers around 1980. During that time, he was a lieutenant, then captain, and finally an assistant chief. He died in 1998.

Francis Sr. was a force and a leader of men. He was friendly, helpful and knowledgeable about any number of subjects. He was also a great father who was very close to his six children. In 1976, his wife tragically died of a brain tumor. At the time his youngest daughter was ten years old. Francis Sr. remained single for many more years, raising the younger children as a single parent.

Francis "Fran" O'Shea, Jr., Chicago Fire Department Paramedic

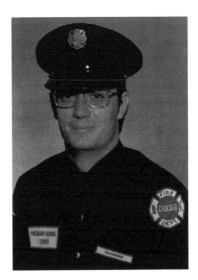

Fran O'Shea Jr as a young CFD Paramedic circa 1975, Courtesy O'Shea family

At the Hoffman Estates Fire Protection District #1, Francis Sr, Francis Jr, and Patrick O'Shea, (Fran's younger brother) were all volunteer firemen. In 1972, they had, collectively, been there for years. Fran Jr. had just turned 21 and had three years on the job already. Stan Zydlo was firing up the EMT and paramedic training and the O'Sheas, without much angst or discussion, decided they were in. They were part of the original 208 volunteers and three of the final 107. They graduated together on December 1, 1972 and went on to stellar careers.

Zydlo, who loved the work effort of the O'Shea trio, pegged them all early as high achievers. Forty plus years later, they did not disappoint. They were the only combination of father/son/siblings in the inaugural group. The "Bull" Kelly blood still percolated.

The Zydlo training was not without its moments of comic relief. Because the firemen worked shifts, Zydlo basically taught double classes on the same subject on back-to-back days. The O'Sheas tried to use this to their advantage, but Zydlo changed it up just enough so that the intelligence getting passed around was not always applicable the next day. For example, everyone figured out really quick that sitting in the front row was likely to get you in Zydlo's gunsights early and often. Pat O'Shea told his brother, so Fran got to class early to sit in the back of the room. Apparently not early enough though because he wound up in the third row, and sure enough Zydlo was lecturing and Fran was doing everything but turning invisible.

Zydlo, of course, immediately jumped on Fran and hammered him. Fran, who already thought Zydlo was a maniac, did not enjoy the wrath of Stan. In time, he understood and came to appreciate the very precise and detailed explanations that were easy to follow.

Fran felt that Zydlo was "pretty crazy," but in a good way that allowed you to flourish under the onslaught. "Dr. Z jammed a lot of information into a short period. It was always simply explained and easy to understand. He would dive down on the floor in a really nice suit and get dirty. He would explain that we would not be treating people who were comfortably lying in bed at a waist high level. He never failed to put it out exactly like he saw it. Stan always stressed to keep it simple and basic. He was one hundred percent right. He never failed to put it out exactly like he saw it."

Fran Jr. and Pat O'Shea continued working at Hoffman Estates until 1974. That is when the Chicago Fire Department finally decided to get some paramedics working the streets. For two years, while Zydlo's guys were racking up big stats and saving lives, City of Chicago citizens were dropping like houseflies in December. When the political masters finally came to their senses, they started to hire paramedics as quickly as they applied. Yet there were a lot of bugs to be worked out and protocols to be put in place; all was not sunshine and moderate breezes.

Many Zydlo-trained medics eventually worked at the CFD. They were known as "*Zydlo Paramedics*." The O'Shea brothers and Elsbeth Miller, the first female paramedic and first woman hired by CFD, a *Zydlo Paramedic*", all worked together in the absolute worst and most violent parts of the city. They were magnificent in the field and, in the best tradition of "Bull" Kelly, a gigantic pain in the ass to their bosses.

One of the earliest and biggest complaints of the "Zydlo medics" was CFD's policy of not allowing paramedics to intubate patients. This was a basic Zydlo tenet and they were losing people because they could not get air into them. Fran O'Shea bitched long and hard about this policy. Outside of the street guys and Elsbeth, no one much cared. Finally, he ran into Stan and told him about it.

Zydlo, who at this point was approaching legend status, blew. He could not believe that his guys, who he personally trained, were being denied this tool that was a game changer in EMS. It saved a lot of lives and Zydlo's world-class temper was reaching volcanic levels when he finally got the CFD's medical director on the phone. He cut right to the chase and without any ceremony lit the medical director up. Basically it went like this:

Zydlo: "Are you fucking people crazy or stupid down there?"

CFD: "Excuse me, Doctor. What did you say?"

Zydlo: You do realize that you are killing people by denying them intubation?"

CFD: "Doctor, we have our own protocols in the city."

Zydlo: "Your protocols are killing people!"

A couple of weeks later, Fran O'Shea was at a training seminar with the medical director Zydlo had chewed on. The medical director figured out real fast that it was O'Shea who was the cause of his sore ass. He had a surprise for Paramedic O'Shea. On the floor was a medical mannequin used for training. Without ceremony or warning, the medical director called Fran to the front of the class and said to him, "Ok, hot shot intubate the patient."

Now O'Shea had not intubated a patient in months, but in the great tradition of "Bull" Kelly, O'Shea grabbed the laryngoscope, tipped the mannequin's head back to a "sniffing position" and intubated the patient in under 15 seconds. He sat down and the medical director paused a second before he said, "Well, I guess you are a *Zydlo trained medic.*"

A few months later, an order came down from CFD headquarters allowing the paramedics to start intubating patients. Shortly thereafter, Zydlo was hired by CFD as a paid medical consultant. CFD may have been a little slow, but they were not brain dead. Somewhere "Bull" and Leo Kelly were tipping a cold one and admiring their grandson's moxie.

Chicago is not anything like most of the suburbs that surround it. The level of violence and the carnage that is non-stop has a quick way of making one feel old. The first responders who work in the trenches do not age gracefully. They get shot at, beat up, and on occasion, killed. It is not a job that promotes a healthy old age and anyone who has worked there for any amount of time begins considering alternative employment about six months into the fray.

The tipping point for Fran O'Shea was when he and his partner got attacked as they walked up to a housing project. For whatever reason, gang members decided to shoot the two paramedics. The two men got behind some cover and were pinned down until the police came to the rescue. It took Fran O'Shea about four years, almost five thousand runs, and a lop-sided gunfight, to pull his trigger. Patrick O'Shea also decided that it was time to go.

Timing is everything. About the time that Fran contemplated a career in carpentry and eight hours of sleep a night one of his bosses at CFD approached Pat and him about leaving CFD and joining him at the Schaumburg, Illinois Fire Department. SFD poached highly qualified studs from the CFD about as fast as they could recruit them. The boss, who was a CFD legend, didn't have to ask twice. Fran and Pat packed their bags and jumped. They were going home.

Schaumburg, Illinois is not Chicago by any stretch of the imagination, but it is not Mayberry, either. It is a busy urban area with all the action one can handle. It has it all, but just in more manageable numbers. The fire department is world class and that's not by accident. It's ten miles northwest of the city of Chicago and O'Hare airport. With almost 75,000 residents, it is a city in every sense of the word with an airport, convention center, and one of the world's largest indoor malls. Its fire department has four stations and 138 sworn personnel who are also paramedics. They have a sophisticated and world class EMS department that is as professional as it gets. It was also one of the original departments in the paramedic program having graduated six members in the inaugural class.

Fran O'Shea did not miss a beat when he went to work at SFD in 1979. He had seen and done it all. He was not going to get surprised and the younger paramedics and fireman thought of him as a legend. He was not yet thirty years old and he was a force. He was old school and people like Zydlo thought of him as a star. He was uncompromising and he knew all the tricks of the job, a fireman's fireman and the keeper of the flame. He was the total package. Predictably, he rose in rank and stature as the years crept by.

Patrick stayed until 2008 when he retired after thirty-six years of service to the brotherhood. He now lives in the Phoenix, Arizona area.

Then there is Timothy O'Shea, Fran's son, "Bull's" great-grandson and Leo's grandson, now a Glenview, Illinois firefighter, just beginning his paramedic training. Timothy is a fifth generation firefighter, bringing his family's collective history to over 120 active years in the fire and paramedic service.

It is now 2016 and Fran O'Shea is the last of the original men still on the job. He has been going at it since 1969 and has been a paramedic since 1973. He has been continually employed as a paramedic/firefighter since 1973---47 years of working in fire departments, 42 years as a full time firefighter and six as a full time paramedic. He made Lieutenant in 1993, which may make him the most senior lieutenant, (23 years) in the United States. He runs his own firehouse and is thinking of retirement because the nine firemen on the Lieutenant list are sick of waiting and have made some noise about "old guys falling off ladders."

He knows he is in the twilight years of this career. He has always worked a second job as a contractor. He paid for his kids' college educations. He compared that to taking two newly-purchased Harley Davidson motorcycles and pushing them off a cliff every year and doing it again four more times. Like his early mentor, Dr. Zydlo, he has heard the end coming. He still loves the job and his guys. He accomplished far more than he ever thought possible. He kept the flame alive and he stayed true to the brotherhood. In the grandest and best traditions of the EMS and fire service, Lt. Francis O'Shea Jr. has not disappointed.

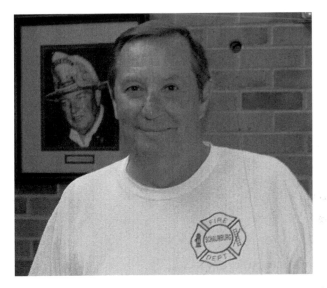

Lt. Fran O'Shea, Scaumburg IL Fire Department, August 2016. Paul Ciolino

In life there are people who talk a lot and a rare few that get things done. Throughout this book we have chronicled some of the stories about folks who get it done. Collectively, they neither seek nor ask for glory or recognition. They simply go out and perform. They do it in ways that civilians could never fully appreciate or understand. None of them could be accused of doing it for the money. They are woefully underpaid. They get old before their time and many never make it long enough to grab that ever elusive pension check.

Many of the people who read this will wonder about why the incompetent, lazy, and stupid that practice this profession were not included here. The answer is really quite simple. Plenty is written about those people who slip by. The personnel who develop drug and alcohol issues and harm the occasional patient are well represented by their attorneys and unions.

The rest usually don't last long. We chose to document what is important and what has not been written about in any meaningful way. We chose to write about the heroes.

It is not all sunshine, puppy dog tails, and champagne in the Ambo. You are talking about alpha male and females working in closely confined spaces under immense pressure. None of these folks fall under the category of "shy and retiring." They are bright, aggressive, and opinionated. They do not suffer fools. They carry the same baggage to work as the rest of us--marital problems, financial woes, etc.---they are not exempt from life's complications.

Yet somehow, they manage to park it when that Ambo rolls out the front door. They forget their differences, their problems, and what an asshole their boss is. They generally perform above and beyond. They do it so often that it has become common. Outside of the firehouse, you are not likely to hear about their frequent miraculous actions. That is how routine it has become and by way of comparison these days the police generally hold a press conference when they don't break a law or get indicted. If they do something spectacular like solve a crime, their department spokesperson will be on TV for the next week at five, six, and ten.

When American Airline jets slammed into the Twin Towers on September 11, 2001, 343 firefighters, including a chaplain, two paramedics and a fire marshal of the New York City Fire Department went into the buildings to do what they do and for their heroic efforts got killed. In addition, eight emergency medical personnel from private ambulance services were killed. Now here is the thing about those men and women: They went into those buildings knowing full well that they might not come out. Who *does* that?

In this instance, sixty police officers were also killed, but generally nobody runs into these disasters like the men and woman who do these jobs and that is the defining DNA that runs through their veins. In general, they know before they get killed that going into that structure, working that accident scene, whatever, may damn well result in their death and a nice fancy funeral. This fact alone separates them from the rest of the general population and this is why Stan Zydlo fought so ferociously for his paramedics and the program.

He knew without question that he would attend a lot of funerals for these warriors. He understood the pain, the grief, and the misery that came with the territory. He was an eyewitness to the Our Lady of the Angels disaster and he knew what was at stake. He was also aware of what these men and woman could accomplish., the second chances they would give people. Just consider the funerals that did *not happen* because of their efforts. These are the things that Zydlo knew and that is what drove him.

The paramedics' collective impact on humanity, their communities, and society in general, can never be measured. His paramedics seldom disappointed Zydlo. He always knew that it would evolve into this. On more than one occasion, Stan talked about these issues and his take was simply this: "Saving lives is something you choose to do or you quit real fast. Do the right thing; do it because you want someone to do it for your family or you. Don't complain; no time for that---just do it and do it right."

A wonderful, very simple, philosophy that has served us all very well for going on five decades now.

CHAPTER NINE

Where the Boys Are

"Men of quality are threatened by women of equality"
–Unknown

It took a while, but it happened. When Dr. Zydlo started the paramedic program with the firemen, there were no women in any of the fire departments. It was 1972 and women had not yet cracked the ranks of one of the last bastions of all-male organizations. Zydlo was concerned, but he always knew that women would have no difficulty in meeting the training standards and eventual licensing requirements. Women had been physicians for decades by the time Stan came around, so for him this was never an issue.

For the women, however, it was not easy. There were no marching bands awaiting their arrival into the fire service. Today, no one blinks when they observe a female paramedic. It is barely newsworthy when a woman is named fire chief in any fire department, no matter how big or small. With these facts in mind, the examination of female paramedics in the early years is historically significant.

Zydlo's initial standards for gaining admittance to the training was that you had to work for a fire department, police department, or ambulance company. In 1972, there were not many women working for those organizations. No sooner had the local media written about this new phenomenon known as the paramedic service than the national media began to write about it. Soon, the international media reprinted or jumped on the story. Prehospital medical applications were completed on the streets and in the homes of America, and the excitement spread like wild fire through the rest of the western world.

Elsbeth's Story

It did not take long for a woman to crack the paramedic ranks. Elsbeth Miller was raised on the east coast in Connecticut. She could fly downhill on skis before she could ride a bike. This would prove to be the foundation for her entry into the relatively new all-boys club known as "paramedics".

For the millions of people who live and ply their trades outside of urban areas where the first paramedics worked, this lack of paramedic service quickly became an enormous gaping hole in the new system. For Elsbeth Miller, then a member of the mostly volunteer U.S. Ski Patrol---expert skiers who responded to injured skiers on the mountains of the world---it was obvious what had to be done.

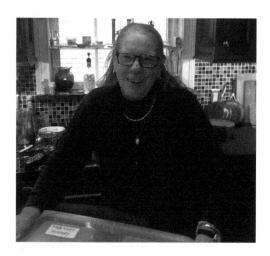

Retired CFD paramedic and 1st ever female paramedic Elsbeth Miller, July 2016.
Paul Ciolino

In tourist areas where skiing was a huge commercial venture, the ski patrol was essential to saving lives and rendering serious first aid. Like any sport that involves a human being traveling at speeds up to sixty, seventy miles an hour, injuries occurred. Often devastating, even life threatening injuries, as well as death, occurred. Mountains are difficult to access and not ambulance friendly. You can't simply whistle an ambulance up there.

Elsbeth Miller knew the moment she heard about Dr. Zydlo and his paramedic program that he was not coming to the mountain any time soon, so she would take herself and the mountain to him. She would become the first woman Stan trained and licensed. Had she gone back to the ski resorts and trails of Connecticut and Vermont, no one would likely have heard of her accomplishment. For anyone who is the "first" in anything, there are special and unique challenges that must be overcome and endured. Fortunately, for the women and the lives they saved throughout the last forty plus years, Elsbeth Miller, like her male colleagues, did in word and deed have the "right stuff".

It is a fact that she was the first licensed female paramedic. It would be difficult to overshadow that accomplishment, but Elsbeth certainly managed to do that when she applied for, and became, the first ever woman hired at the Chicago Fire Department (CFD). Eclipsing that accomplishment, she was the only female paramedic to work for, and eventually retire from, the CFD after thirty-eight years of service. Like her first mentor, Stan Zydlo, Elsbeth Miller would also reach that lofty and Olympian worthy platform known as *legend*.

Elsbeth's Story

Sitting in Elsbeth's gourmet kitchen in her modest home on the northwest side of Chicago in late 2015, I quickly got a sense of how much iron is left in her spine. Like her male brethren, she has seen too much death and carnage. She has abused her body and soul like few other women in history. She left it all out there in the streets, alleys, and housing projects of Chicago and now she looks like more of a cookie-making Grandma than a hard case paramedic/firefighter. Like Zydlo, though, the body went long before the heart and spirit. Several job-related surgeries and injuries beat her up pretty good, but her spirit and her whip-smart personality have not lost a beat.

Elsbeth Thraikill-Miller was a young ski junkie who lived on the slopes and mountains of New England. Her parents had moved to Barrington, Illinois where her father was a high level executive with Alberto Culver, a company that produced hair and skin care beauty products.

Elsbeth was finishing high school and living alone in Vermont in the family home and skiing, playing tennis and having a good time. She was fourteen years old when she became a member of the volunteer U.S. Ski Patrol and finished EMT training while still living on the east coast. She was an action junkie and high level athlete in every sense of the word.

Her parents, friends with a newspaper publisher in Barrington, Illinois, had closely followed the brand new paramedic program initiated by Stan Zydlo. They told Elsbeth about it, and she took about five minutes to decide to hop on the first thing smoking and come to Chicago to let Dr. Zydlo know she wanted in---now.

Stan Zydlo had a policy that you had to be working for a fire or police department before he would let you in his new paramedic program. After deciding that the United States Ski Patrol in Vermont was close enough to being a fire department, Zydlo simply said "Go back home and pack your shit." Thus, Elsbeth was immediately admitted to the paramedic program. On occasion, it is convenient, and wise, to be a benevolent dictator.

On June 25, 1974, Elsbeth completed and passed the paramedic test. Zydlo thought she was an exceptional student and would have no problem with the job. The problem was that no fire department had any female employees. The other thirty-two graduates in her class had departments to go back to. Nineteen-year-old Elsbeth was on a raft with no destination in sight. Vermont was looking good and she was sick of the non-skiing flat surfaces of the Midwest. Like most youthful, Type A personalities, patience was in short supply.

It's important to remember that Zydlo's paramedic program was still in its infancy, but fire departments across the country were stirring and waking up fast. Everyone wanted to copy Zydlo's model. The days of the nurses and doctor's lobbies politicking against the paramedics were over. The consortium of fire departments that started the original program had evolved to a well-oiled lifesaving machine. Zydlo's paramedics were the gold standard that everyone wanted. They were absolutely rocking it.

There was no script and no internet. There was no woman before her. There was certainly no support group who could coach and advise her through the hiring, testing, and application process. She had no clout and zero political sponsorship. She was nineteen years old, unaware of exactly where the city of Chicago was, except she knew she had to drive east to get there. She was so far out of her element it was almost laughable.

She was in Room 105 of the ancient five-story city hall building on LaSalle Street at the Chicago Fire Department's administration offices being interviewed by Deputy Fire Chief Dick Albright, who would later succeed Commissioner Robert Quinn. Today, this would be akin to the vice-president of the United States interviewing a kid for a Secret Service job. Albright was in charge of putting together a paramedic unit for the CFD. It was late 1974 and the CFD was way behind Zydlo's initial paramedic program. Chicago Mayor Richard J. Daley was not happy. He ran the city like a South American dictator and would continue to run it like that until he died in the back of a CFD ambulance on December 20, 1976.

For now, though, he had waved his pinkie ring at the Fire Commissioner and said, "Make it happen."

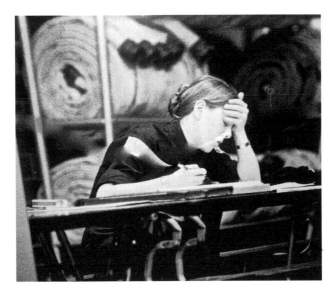

CFD Paramedic Elsbeth Miller writing a report. Circa 1976. Courtesy Elsbeth Miller.

Like another long ago ruler named Julius Caesar, Daley was not interested in how his orders were carried out. He never wanted to give an order twice, but if he did that was usually the last day of employment for whoever ignored the first order.

Complicating this paramedic business was the fact that the CFD had never in its entire history hired a woman firefighter. Commissioner Quinn and Deputy Chief Albright were old school. They liked their women at home baking cookies and minding the children. They very much disliked this edict, but being very experienced in the political realities of Chicago and the very real possibility of being *former* Commissioner and *former* Deputy Chief they did not screw around.

Elsbeth Miller was unaware of all these Machiavellian plots swirling about city hall and naïve enough to believe she had a legitimate shot at getting a paramedic job. She had zero political agenda. She was not a feminist in the truest definition of the word, and she absolutely had no cause celeb except getting an opportunity to become a paramedic. Albright wanted to know one thing. "Obviously you're a female. How do you expect us to accommodate you?" Elsbeth looked him straight in the eye and simply said, "I expect absolutely nothing."

One month later she received a letter from the CFD that began, "Dear Sir". She skipped the 'Sir' part and went right to the part that told her to report to the Fire Department Academy to take a physical agility test. To qualify for the fire department, she had to pass the physical fitness test and there were no exceptions. There was no explanation as to what this test would entail.

A few weeks later, Elsbeth showed up for the test. There was a welcoming committee of two CFD personnel officers present just to observe the test and to make sure that Elsbeth didn't receive any breaks. There were no preliminary pep talks. There was no warm up. Elsbeth had not worked out or exercised in months. She could not have been more physically unprepared if she had tried.

She was about 5'3" tall and maybe weighed a hundred and ten pounds. The next smallest person in the group outweighed her by forty pounds. Most of the men weighed at least fifty pounds more. Some of them a hundred pounds or even more. There wasn't a female within twenty miles. Elsbeth had them all exactly where she wanted them.

Lying below a five-story metal open staircase was an ambulance stretcher with a plywood box containing a simulated Life Pack II on top of it. Sitting on top of the five-story structure was a mannequin that weighed one hundred and eighty pounds. It was all dead weight---and in a bathtub.

Elsbeth had breezed through all the other tests. She was slaying this thing. But this was the man-eater part of the test. This was the one-way ticket back to the ski slopes. She watched guys drop like flies on this portion. A crowd had developed and it was eerily quiet. She had to get the stretcher and plywood box up the five-story structure with a partner. When (if) she got there she had to muscle the 180-pound dead weight out of the bathtub by herself and onto the stretcher; then, with a "partner", muscle the whole thing back down the stairs intact.

All of this was timed and not one person there believed that this 5'3", buck ten, doe-eyed nineteen-year-old beauty could do it. At this point in CFD's history, no female had even attempted it. Men, especially second and third generation firefighter candidates, had failed this test for years after they had trained for months. There was never a doubt and don't you know it, Elsbeth smoked this thing and no one could believe what they had just witnessed. Elsbeth was gassed and feeling more relieved than accomplished. She looked downright tiny, especially next to the men, many of whom were in great shape. But she had something none of them had--- thighs that looked like cut granite. Her strength was in her lower body. She didn't just look good; she was a damn beast. Pounding those ski slopes since preschool had turned her into a physical specimen that bordered on professional athlete territory.

As with everything in the long, torrid, corrupt history of the City of Chicago, there was a hitch. Although fifty or sixty independent witnesses had watched Elsbeth pass the physical test, there was a problem in the form of Deputy Chief Jim Harper, the newly-appointed head of paramedic services. He wasn't buying into this girl firefighter/paramedic stuff for one second. He arrived at the academy after Elsbeth had passed all the tests. Though informed that their lone female applicant had just passed the test, Harper was unimpressed and told the test proctor that he didn't believe it. He ordered her to take the stretcher test again. Not tomorrow, not next week. Right then.

In a career filled with firsts, Elsbeth Miller took the test again. That made her the first applicant ever to do the test twice in the same day after having successfully passed it the first time. Had Dr. Zydlo been present, he might have gutted Harper right on the spot. Zydlo wasn't there and no person present would take on the high ranking deputy chief.

For a second time in less than an hour, Elsbeth hit the proverbial grand slam with two outs in the ninth and the bases loaded. She scrambled up and down those stairs and, in the grand tradition of those Zydlo-trained medics, she smoked that test for a second time with a better time than the first one. Harper watched silently, turned on his heel and left without a congratulatory word. Elsbeth received a second letter giving her a report date for the Fire Department Academy. They were still "Dear Sir'ing" her, but it didn't offend her in the least. She never looked backward again.

Being nineteen has its advantages. You're not yet hardened to the realities and disappointments of life. You believe that most people are good; they are fair and they are honest. Mostly though, you are not from Chicago and you still might believe in all these niceties, but reality is starting to set in. The bogus re-test Elsbeth was forced to endure was just the beginning of her getting "Chicagoized". The disappointments would continue for many of her thirty-eight years of service and would only get more complicated and more Machiavellian in nature.

Reporting on November 29, 1974 to the fire academy with forty-nine male candidates was not as bad as she might have anticipated after the Harper incident. She found her instructors, almost all old timers, to be knowledgeable and friendly. Most treated her with respect and dignity. She felt very welcomed. There was little talk of her being the first female hired and even fewer issues regarding her being the first female paramedic. Reflecting many years later, Elsbeth felt that the instructors, and most of her early bosses, treated her like a daughter or granddaughter. For the most part, she was welcomed into the brotherhood without any drama. She was happy and liked everything she learned. This firefighter/paramedic stuff was right in her wheelhouse.

She graduated without any fanfare. There was no press and no one mentioned that Elsbeth had just cracked a hundred plus years of tradition, as well as the all-boys club, and was now a sworn firefighter/paramedic before she was twenty years old. This was rarified air and the Chicago Fire Department had not one clue what to do with her. They had to waive the height and weight requirements for her and there were zero bathroom or separate sleeping arrangements available for women. The CFD members have a saying they break out when they are feeling a little abused, "*150 years of tradition uninterrupted by progress.*"

She was blissfully ignorant of all the behind the scenes angst and the potential political disaster should this little experiment involving her fail. By and large her male colleagues wanted her to succeed. Their wives on the other hand, had the knives out. Almost to a person they wanted her gone. This hot little 'chickie' was not going to "break up my happy home." Let's face it, firemen have never been confused with saints and eunuchs. Firehouses are testosterone driven places filled with good looking, manly men who *really like women*…a lot. Putting a good-looking, smoking hot, twenty-year-old beauty amongst them was just a little too tempting for many of them. The wives, well, they did not know Elsbeth, but they sure knew their husbands.

There were a lot of meetings and a lot of brainpower spent on where to assign Elsbeth. The CFD has had at various times, give or take a few, one hundred firehouses and five thousand sworn personnel. The city is divided into eight districts. It's the second largest fire department in the United States and they stay busy. You would think they could easily find a spot for one female firefighter.

She was assigned to O'Hare airport in the far northwest corner of the city. It is about as far as you can get from downtown and still actually be in the city of Chicago. At that time, O'Hare was the busiest airport in the world, handling more than 37.8 million passengers on almost 695,000 flights.[12] It was a great assignment because she was always busy there. She had excellent bosses who were "old school". They really wanted her to succeed and do well. There were zero issues concerning her gender.

Elsbeth describes her time at O'Hare as "being raised and getting taught how to be a fireman." This is where she was drilled about the code of conduct and the brotherhood of which she was now a member. If there was any animosity about her being the first woman in CFD, it was overridden by her colleagues' efforts to raise her right. "I was raised like any other young fireman and it was never about my sex," she recalled.

Historically, the timing was perfect. Elsbeth came on the job when the CFD was transitioning from the old days to the modern era. The older members of the department had all this institutional knowledge and their time left on the job was coming to a close. She learned from men who had mostly come on the job right after World War II and the Korean War. Most of them were present for the 1958 fire at the Our Lady of the Angels grammar school that had killed 92 children and three Catholic nuns. Many people would consider these firemen "dinosaurs" past their prime. Elsbeth knew immediately their knowledge was critical for her survival and any future success she might enjoy.

It didn't take very long for Elsbeth to find out about the dark side of a public service job. At the fire academy the lectures covered what benefits the paramedic/firefighters would receive. The paramedics were told they were in the same retirement system as the firemen. But they were *not* in that system. They were told they were under the same medical and disability benefits as the firemen, but they were, in fact, in a different system.

These, as well as other promises made to them, came boiling to a head very early on. It happened when another paramedic was injured on the job. When the paramedics learned they were not covered under the same rules as the firemen and had been lied to about a number of issues, they decided to organize. They did this by forming the American Association of Trauma Specialists. Elsbeth was an officer and secretary-treasurer.

This association was the prelude to becoming a union. When they insisted on meeting with the city officials to address their grievances, some very serious trouble started. On October 14, 1975, the city fired Pat Stevens, Mickey Dunn, and Elsbeth Miller for bogus and made-up charges. Coincidently, all three were senior officers in the newly-formed paramedic association. Elsbeth had not yet been on the job for a year and her career was over before it had barely begun. She was devastated, but she and her friends were also prepared, as well as determined.

Elsbeth, Dunn, and Stevens immediately filed an 8.9-million-dollar lawsuit against the city and Fire Commissioner Quinn in federal court in the Northern District Court of Illinois on the day they were fired. Their attorney, Kim Denkewalter, was able to get an emergency hearing in front of Federal Judge Prentice Marshall on the same day. Marshall, like all federal judges, had a lifetime appointment. The city held absolutely no sway over him. He had watched the City of Chicago run roughshod over its employees for years. He knew bullshit when he smelled it and he just lit the city up. Without delay, he granted an injunction against Quinn, the fire department and the City. He ordered all three paramedics back to work the same day. The three of them did not so much as miss a shift.

In a number of firsts in her life, Elsbeth was also the first female paramedic to be fired by CFD and the first female employee to ever successfully sue the city. The firsts were racking up at breakneck speed and she was not yet twenty-one-years old. If any firemen still doubted a woman could do the job, they didn't doubt her integrity and unwillingness to take any shit from anyone. Word of what she had done quickly spread through the whole department. Who was this broad?

Within a very short time, the City caved in and Elsbeth and the men were given all the benefits originally promised. The city that was used to having its way forever with its employees was not happy. It was the dawn of a new age in Chicago and Elsbeth Miller not only had a view, she had a seat at the table.

All of these issues were building blocks for Elsbeth. She had been on the job for just over a year when the *Chicago Sun Times* published an article on December 7, 1975 titled, "Paramedics save life of executive".[13] The article featured a picture of Elsbeth and the caption underneath read, "Her team did it"; "Elsbeth Thraikill (Miller) the senior paramedic on the team that saved the life of Robert Vaughn.". It would be the first of dozens of lives she saved in the next thirty-eight plus years.

After the lawsuit and its bad ending for the city, Elsbeth settled into her job and the life of a paramedic. She was well-liked and respected by her peers and loved her work. It even got to a point that it was far more exciting than racing down the side of a mountain. She was exposed to, and worked in, the worst neighborhoods and assignments. She lost count of the number of gunshot victims she treated. Other female paramedics were hired and did well on the job.

In August of 1979, Elsbeth was promoted to 'Paramedic in Charge'. She was beginning to think about starting a family and having children. She got married in 1980 to another CFD fireman. They had two children, a son David and a daughter Morgan. Both children were extremely smart and attended Chicago's famed Latin School, which is generally reserved for the children of Chicago's wealthier, more connected, citizens. Elsbeth was neither wealthy nor connected, but she came from money and understood the game. At the Latin social functions, Elsbeth would occasionally show up in uniform and get the look of "Hey, the help goes around the back" look. Big mistake. One does not make that mistake with Elsbeth a second time. The marriage did not last, but that seemed to have little effect on the children as they went on to stellar academic and professional careers. The University of Chicago, ranked as the fourth best university in the United States, has been quietly giving a very few scholarships a year to one or two children of the Chicago Police and Fire Departments. A school that charges over sixty-four thousand dollars a year in tuition, room, and board is way out of reach for any children of a public servant. The school only accepts about eight percent of the people who apply, so this is a real game changer for anyone fortunate enough to attend. Receiving and winning a scholarship from U of C is akin to winning the multi-state Powerball lottery.

Elsbeth's son, David, won the prestigious scholarship after he graduated from Lane Tech High School in Chicago. Following graduation from the University of Chicago, he went to Stanford University and earned his Ph.D. Today, he is a physics professor at the University of Chicago, specializing in Experimental High Energy Particle Physics.

Elsbeth's daughter, Morgan, attended Lane Tech High School, as well, and graduated from the University of Illinois at Chicago. She is currently employed as an Intensive Care R.N. at a large Chicago hospital. She and her husband are expecting their first child.

Apparently Elsbeth does not do anything small.

On February 14, 1980, after years of labor strife and broken promises from the City of Chicago, the CFD firemen went on strike. Ninety-six percent of the fire department (96%) sworn personnel walked off the job and the gloves came off. Prior to this date, the firemen had always had a very tenuous relationship with the city over a myriad of labor problems. The single biggest issue for the firemen was staffing and manpower issues.

There were also serious issues involving training, outdated equipment, and assignments. These are all very legitimate issues, but for the firemen the really big, nuclear bomb issue was a broken promise. In 1978, a relatively unknown, minor political figure named Jane Byrne decided to run for mayor in Chicago. A Democrat, she was in the fight of her political life in a primary election against a sitting Democratic mayor named Michael Bilandic.

Bilandic had been a hand-picked successor to Mayor Richard M. Daley and was the odds on favorite to get re-elected. Byrne was desperate and went hat in hand to the members of the CFD. The CFD is no stranger to Chicago politics and was well-versed in the fragile and potentially dangerous ramifications of getting involved in an election between political heavyweights who controlled their very life. Getting involved on the wrong side (translate loser) could set the organization back years. Nevertheless, the CFD listened to Byrne's rap and bought in.

Byrne, a Northsider (all Chicagoans know you can't trust a Northsider) was endorsed by the rank and file of the CFD. They endorsed her prior to the primary and Byrne, in turn, unequivocally pledged her support as mayor should she win the election. She won by a narrow margin and promptly reneged, (the Southside firemen had been right) on her promises to the CFD and this caused the most serious labor dispute in the history of Chicago.

The core issue was Byrne had promised to sign a negotiated contract with the CFD recognizing their unionization and collective bargaining rights. Byrne who was a hard drinking, profane, Irish politician from the old school thought that she could bully and do whatever she felt like doing to the membership of the CFD. It was a huge tactical error on her part and the firemen went after her with everything they had. The general public was overwhelmingly in favor of the firemen in this instance. Chicago has always been a union town and Byrne overestimated her popularity by committing the cardinal sin of politics, which is, simply, do not fight with the police or fire departments. If you do, you had better pick the *right* fight.

By this time, Elsbeth was also a pretty hardcore union activist on the part of the paramedics. At this point in her life she had been playing hardball for years with the pols and she was not the same young, innocent New Englander who was naïve in the ways of power and senior management. She was now a true Chicagoan who explicitly knew the rules of Street Fighting Politics 101.

From February 14 through March 7, 1980, Elsbeth and her fellow firemen/paramedics went out on strike and did not work. The fire department's response was to rush recruits out of the fire academy early and hire eight hundred people who crossed the picket line. The bad feelings over the strikebreakers last to this day.

As for the strikers, they were not militant enough to just allow fires to do what fires do. In fact, *"As soon as there was a fire or something where somebody was injured, we would jump in our personal cars, drive to that area. If we had a fire, we would go in and grab the hose lines from the [firefighters who] crossed the picket lines. There was like 1,000 people who came on [to break the strike]. They did not know which end of the hose was which."*

"We'd go inside, put the fire out, make sure everybody was safe. Then we would hand all the tools back, go back to the firehouse and hold our picket signs...We owned our own fire coats and helmets. But a lot of us were just in blue jeans and gym shoes running into the fire...We were not gonna let someone die in our neighborhood because of the strike."[14]

Mayor Richard M. Daley was quoted at a meeting in October 1976, saying *"Even though you never got a contract out of me, you better get one when I'm gone."*[15] Once again the firemen brought the city to its knees when they got almost every benefit for which they went on strike. Elsbeth Miller was right in the middle of it.

During the next several years, Elsbeth worked paramedic assignments all over the City of Chicago. She worked some nice quiet, affluent areas of the city. She was an instructor at the CFD Fire Academy for a couple of years. She also worked in the absolute worst parts of the city. She worked in Humboldt Park for over fifteen years where she and her team would dodge bullets while trying to save gunshot and stabbing victims of the notorious Latin Kings street gang. She worked in Lincoln Park, a very affluent part of the city. She also worked in the notorious Cabrini Green housing project, which was so violent that Mayor Jane Byrne moved into it for ten days during the time she was mayor. Albeit she moved in with a dozen badass Chicago Police officers, she still moved in. It got pretty quiet with the massive police presence temporarily assigned there. It was so violent that the Chicago and national media began referring to Chicago as, "Beirut on the Lake". Elsbeth worked those projects every day and she and her partners did it without the benefit of CPD bodyguards.

In 1995, Elsbeth was promoted to Ambulance Commander and she still worked the streets. The Ambulance Commander rank was equal to the rank of captain. Elsbeth was at the height of her paramedic powers. She had worked in every part of the city to include Bridgeport where the former Mayor Daleys and Mayor Bilandic had lived. It was a nice quiet assignment, but it was not half as active as what she was familiar with. Elsbeth does not do easy. She managed to get transferred back to the west side where the real action was and, in 2006, she received her last CFD promotion when she became Field Chief. It was a big title and a big job. She was responsible for four battalions of paramedics and all that went with that. She often responded to anywhere in the city and was involved in every conceivable tragedy that a public servant can work.

In 1995, woman paramedics were no longer an oddity or an experiment. Elsbeth was an ambulance commander and she was a force. She was into her second decade in this business and was, without question, a legend. Peeking under the tent one would think that Elsbeth could not have avoided seeing everything that the violent streets of Chicago could toss her way.

But, on a warm summer day on Chicago's west side, in the Humboldt Park neighborhood, she and her partner, another woman paramedic named Mercedes Mora, were about to encounter a situation that would tax their considerable skills. The two women, who were regular partners, prided themselves on never asking for help. They had not seen or worked a situation they could not handle.

They were working on Ambulance Number 3 and Engine 43 when they got a call about a man bleeding on the street. They proceeded to Pulaski and Fullerton Avenues where they found a significant blood trail, but no man. They got out of the ambulance, grabbed their stretcher chair, and followed the blood trail. Down the sidewalk, to a stoop of a two-flat apartment building, up the stoop stairs, into the vestibule, up the narrow rickety stairs as the blood trail gets more pronounced with every step. The entire stairwell, walls, and hallway are covered in blood. Just when they think it can't get any worse---it does.

When Elsbeth and Mercedes walked into the second floor apartment, the place looked like a slaughterhouse. There was blood everywhere and laying in the middle of it is a thirtyish young man attired only in a pair of nylon running shorts. He's a big, good-looking kid who weighs around 200 pounds. He's barely conscious and covered in blood. The paramedics find a small puncture wound, about an inch and half long, by his femoral artery. He has no other injuries. But they know an adult male this size would have approximately 10 pints of blood in his body. Elsbeth does the math in her head as she walks up to the victim. She realizes that he is about as bled out as a human can get.

Dr. Zydlo, who always preached that the paramedics would quite often be dealing with people on the worst day of their life, proved to be spot on in this case. The young guy at this point had about a two percent chance of surviving his current circumstance.

There are three spots that you do not want to be bleeding if you are injured. The worst is an aorta bleed by the heart. The second is the jugular vein in your neck. The third is your femoral artery in your leg/groin area. There is simply not a lot of time if you get cut in one of those areas.

Elsbeth and Mercedes struggled with this guy. They could barely stand as they slid and slopped around in the blood. There was nothing to hold onto. Two Chicago Police Patrolmen from the Shakespeare District sauntered into the room and could not believe their eyes. They had never seen so much blood in one spot. Elsbeth knew in this instance that they would not be much help. She later recalled that the Shakespeare District police were magnificent---the best in the city---but "they don't do blood very well." In a herculean moment, the two women finally got the kid loaded onto the stretcher chair and down they went, slip-slopping through all the blood. They wheeled him to the back of the ambulance and put him on the long stretcher. They cleared the scene in six minutes.

The second they got him secured in the back, they dropped a 14-gauge needle in each arm and pumped fluids into him. They didn't bother with his blood pressure as at this point he was not bleeding--there was no blood left in him. They give him 100% pure oxygen, but can't get the IV fluid in him fast enough.

Mercedes jumped in the front of the ambulance and off they went. They are off to Illinois Masonic Hospital on the north side. They were several miles away and in the back of the ambulance things were not going well at all. Illinois Masonic has a crack team of trauma surgeons. Elsbeth and Mercedes realize that if they can deliver this guy alive, he might have a chance.

Mercedes ran the bus like Helio Castroneves at the Indianapolis 500, while Elsbeth tried to figure out how to get the necessary fluids into the victim. She remembered a conversation with Dr. Sheldon "Shelly" Maltz, a trauma surgeon at Illinois Masonic, a few weeks prior. Dr. Maltz had told Elsbeth that you could only get about two liters of fluids into an individual in the time allowed in the ambulance. So Elsbeth knew two things: two liters would not cut it, and Dr. Maltz, brilliant surgeon that he was, had not studied "street medicine".

Once again. Elsbeth worked the problem out and the numbers looked like shit. She had to get more fluids into the victim. Then it hit her. She grabbed the blood pressure cups and wrapped them around each of the 1000cc bags of saline. She pumped up the cuffs as tight as she could get them and, don't you know, those blood pressure cups squeezed the IV bags, turning them into a high-pressure hose. Now she was cooking. The saline shot into the victim's body about as fast as mechanically possible.

The victim was still breathing when Elsbeth and Mercedes delivered him to the ER where the trauma team grabbed him and wheeled him up to emergency surgery. They later learned that the victim survived and, after four long months at the hospital, he finally went back home.

This was perhaps one of the greatest saves in the history of paramedics and yet until now few people have known about it.

Elsbeth and Mercedes were all about saving lives. They didn't much care about the why or how. They understood, like all of their brethren in this business, sometimes you just had to be extraordinary in the performance of your duties.

They didn't get recognized on this day for their heroic efforts. They didn't even get a free cup of coffee. But as one of the cops who was on the scene that day said later, "Man, if you get fucked up in the street you'd better pray these two broads show up."

For Elsbeth and Mercedes, those kinds of remarks were reward enough.

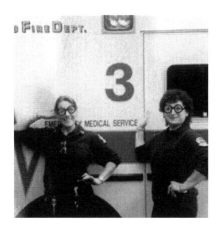

CFD Paramedic's Elsbeth Miller and Mercedes Mora, circa 1988. Courtesy Elsbeth Miller.
Ambulance Commander Elsbeth Miller (left)
Paramedic Mercedes Mora (right)

When the Twin Towers came down on September 11, 2001 in New York City, Elsbeth was one of the high-ranking delegation members of CFD who went to NYC to represent the CFD at dozens of funerals of the murdered NYFD members. She has described it as one of the most difficult things she has ever done.

On December 29, 2012, Elsbeth Miller retired after thirty-eight years of service to the CFD and the City of Chicago. She left it all out there on the street and as she reflects back on this life she feels blessed and fortunate. When she showed up on Dr. Zydlo's door step in 1974 and pretty much demanded to become a paramedic, Zydlo knew this was the woman who would become a legend. She did not disappoint.

She also became what the oldtimers at O'Hare foresaw when the first CFD female hire and paramedic showed up there in 1975. She became, and still is today, a *Firemen's Fireman/Paramedic*. For Elsbeth Miller there is no higher compliment.

For any young person looking for a hero and a historic figure to look up to, look no further. Elsbeth Miller is right here in front of you.

CHAPTER TEN

"The Duke of Austin"

*"We make a living by what we get, but we
make a life by what we give."*
–Winston Churchill

America is great because of its big ideas and even bigger accomplishments. The winning of two world wars, the landing of men on the moon, the greatest economy the world has ever known, the biggest automobile industry, the biggest steel industry, gas and oil exploration, exploring Mars, Waffle House, and medical "break throughs", such as the polio vaccine, and the list goes on and on. All of these successes have been heavily documented and written about.

What generally is not written about anymore is the success and the lifesaving efforts of America's paramedics. The reasons are many. Frankly, as a country we are spoiled. We are apathetic. We very much take for granted that when someone is badly injured, shot, stabbed, run over by a vehicle, or suffering a major cardiac event, we just know for certain that a highly-trained and proficient paramedic and a several hundred-thousand-dollar ambulance is going to come save our life, generally within six minutes or so.

Considering Chicago's record on corruption, it is a miracle that any agency runs efficiently. Since 1972, seventy-nine (79) elected officials have been convicted of corruption. Three governors, twenty other state officials, fifteen state legislators, one mayor, three other city officials, twenty-seven aldermen, and nineteen Cook County judges have been found guilty of, or pleaded to, criminal activity before a court. That is a state wide total of 105, but the City of Chicago leads everyone else with seventy-nine convicted felons.[16]

In the eye of this storm is the Chicago Fire Department which seems mostly unaffected by the dysfunction in the corridors of government. In a city with a population of 2,722,389 and another 40 million annual visitors, the fire department maintains approximately 75 ambulances. They cover an area of 237 square miles. There are over five million 911 calls a year in the city. The Fire Department alone on average handles three-thousand 911 calls *a day*. By comparison, Houston has almost five-hundred-thousand less people then Chicago, but has 88 ambulances. They also have about half as many homicides as Chicago.

By November 2, 2015, four hundred and eighteen people had been murdered in Chicago proper. That is just in ten months. What the headlines and politicians don't talk about very often is the total number of people shot. If the first number in this paragraph does not grab your attention, this one should. Two thousand, five hundred and fifty-eight (2,558) additional people were shot in that time period.

They survived in large part because the Chicago Fire Department paramedics are perhaps in today's world, one of the best collective group of paramedics that has ever bounced around the potholes and speed bumps of Chicago's increasingly broke ass city.

The Chicago Fire Department's paramedic program started in 1974, almost a full two years after Zydlo sent out his first class of licensed paramedics. Chicago can be maddeningly slow like that. Tony Scipione and Gunther Kettenbeil were the first two paramedics hired by the CFD.[17] When they retired together in 2012 after 34 years, they left behind storied careers and a standard of excellence, bravery, and service to their paramedic brethren.

The biggest reason that those 2,500 plus victims survived was because of the heroic efforts of those paramedics to get them to a trauma center breathing and having a fighting chance of getting first class treatment from teams of very experienced trauma personnel who certainly deserve credit, as well. Lest we forget, if victims don't make it there alive, there is no treatment and that is where this episode begins.

It is worth telling because forty-five years after Zydlo started the paramedic program the historical record needed a bridge to today and with that in mind the author decided to suck it up and go hang out with the big boys. Getting permission to do so was not so much difficult as it was interesting. A whole series of emails and phone calls were required, but at the end of the day the bosses at the CFD were totally cooperative and accommodating. They placed very few restrictions on me and once the barn door was open, it was wide open.

The west side of Chicago is a combat zone in every sense of the word. There are no tourists here. There are no fine dining experiences to be had unless you count "Mom's BBQ" or "Uncle Remus Fried Chicken". The Chamber of Commerce does not tout the area as a business haven. Unless they are buying heroin, the 40 million tourists who show up annually never go to Austin. There is a lot of business going on, but it is the business of violence, drugs, gangs, and despair.

Chicago is a city of neighborhoods. Within the city there are at least two hundred neighborhoods. They have names like Bridgeport, Archer Heights, Bronzeville, Beverly, etc. Some of them are named after prominent

citizens, or main streets that run through them or even the sexual preference of the majority of its residents, i.e. "Boystown".

Race, ethnicity, economics, and religion all play a part in who lives
where. Race is generally the biggest factor. There is nowhere in the city of
Chicago that is more poor, more African American, or more violent, than
the west side's Austin neighborhood.

By raw data, Austin consistently has the most homicides in just
about any reporting period. It is the largest by population of the city's sev-
enty-seven officially defined community areas.[18] There are approximately
98,514 souls jammed into a 7.16 square mile area.

Up through the 1960's, Austin had an overwhelmingly white, fairly
affluent population. The 1960 census pegged the white population at
99.83%. Today those numbers are reversed. The African American population is at 85.1%, Hispanic, 8.85%, and white at 4.43%.

The unemployment rate is reported at a ridiculous 21%. In reality, it's
probably closer to 50%. 27% of its households live below the poverty level
and the per capita income is $15,920. In short, there is not a lot to cheer
about in Austin and the misery level of its residents does not appear to be
going anywhere but down.

There are no vacations, weekends off, or down time for crime in
Austin. There were 141 violent crimes, 6 homicides, 5 sexual assaults, 28
assaults, 48 batteries, and 54 robberies. There were 267 property crimes,
180 thefts, 36 burglaries, 47 auto thefts and 4 arsons. There were 417 quality of life crimes, 125 criminal damage, 268 narcotics, and 24 prostitution
arrests. Now you might be saying to yourself, "Well that's not too bad". If
it were for the year it might not be, but those stats are for a 30-day period
from September 24, 2015 through October 24, 2015.[19]

It is in this bleak, violent, Hiroshima type atmosphere that Chicago
Fire Department Ambulance Commander/Paramedic Jay DiGiovanni

plies his trade. As you might have guessed by Jay's last name he is not an African American. He is not a resident of Austin. He doesn't own a liquor store there. He could work anywhere he wants. You might be asking yourself by now (be honest), why in the hell would this highly qualified, very educated, rock star paramedic, white guy, be working in perhaps the most dangerous plot of real estate in the world? Why would he risk getting shot or killed for *"these people"* who are clearly hell bent on killing each other and anyone else who may get in the way of a stray bullet? Perhaps because as the Old School Italians would have said Jay was *la cosa vera*, the real thing, with *"la stoffa giusta,"* the right stuff.

These activities are what Zydlo imagined happening when he thought this up. DiGiovanni is precisely the type of person Zydlo envisioned doing this work. Race, creed, religion, sexual preference, means exactly zero shits to Jay DiGiovanni. In the small circumscribed world of the Chicago Fire Department, Jay DiGiovanni is famous for his skills and lifesaving abilities. He can have his pick of assignments.

Yet he stays in Austin and all he really cares about is: "Man, I hope I can pull this dude/dudette out of it long enough to get him/her to the ER."

He doesn't care about dude's insurance status, race, gang affiliation, or criminal background. He's there to save dude's life and he will not let anything or anyone interfere in that quest. This is who he is and all the background noise that most people hear, well, DiGiovanni is listening to something entirely different than the rest of us mere mortals. He gets it done and he just might get it done as well as anyone who ever did this job. This is partly why Jay DiGiovanni is the *Duke of Austin.*

DiGiovanni is the classic overachiever. He received his bachelor and master's degrees from Chicago's prestigious Loyola University in psychology and counseling psychology. His thesis was on stress in firefighters. His certifications were in advanced cardiac life support, advanced burn life support, the list goes on and on. He is the 21st Century version of the Renaissance man. Yet when he is on the street and responding to all sorts of death and mayhem, he is everyman. He is unassuming and friendly. He takes charge. He makes decisions quickly and cleanly. He does not hesitate. There is not even a hint of wasted motion.

It is an interesting study in poise and leadership and in the time you have spent reading this DiGiovanni, has probably saved another life. It's about this time you're wondering why is this guy working for the City of Chicago when he should be running it? Why indeed?

Mike Kuryla: Chicago Fire Department, Fireman and Paramedic

Mike Kuryla can't remember when he was not in a firehouse. He was literally thrown into the business the old-fashioned way. He was born into it. Mike's father was a career firefighter and just recently retired after 39 years on the department with 22 years as chief of Hillside, Illinois. The next day he became chief of the neighboring town of Berkeley, Illinois's Fire Department.

Mike is 33 years old and has been a fireman or paramedic his entire professional life. For the last three years he has manhandled a high tech half-million-dollar, four-ton Chicago Fire Department ambulance through the Austin combat zone on the west side of Chicago. Prior to that he was an Oak Brook Terrace, Illinois fireman. This is a recurring theme in the CFD. The CFD considers the affluent suburban fire departments their Triple A club. "Kid, go pay your dues on the farm club. We'll bring you up when you're a little more seasoned." An analogy that the suburbs might disagree with, but there are a lot of former suburban guys working at CFD.

Kuryla's affect is pretty unremarkable. He looks like "Mario" in the Mario Brothers' video game. The guy with the stash and big white gloves. You would not give him a second look. Average build, bad mustache, balding, to say the least not a fashion plate. To be frank, at first blush he doesn't look like he's all that bright. He'd be a great stickup guy because only his wife or mom would recognize him a second time.

This is why first impressions are often vastly overrated. Mike Kuryla is exceptionally bright. He is driven and dedicated. There is a lot under the hood. He does not suffer fools, but he is kind, considerate and professional. He's a team player, well-liked and respected by his colleagues. He keeps his head down, mouth shut, and does his job quickly and competently. He is a perfect complement to his boss and partner, Jay DiGiovanni.

Ambulance #15

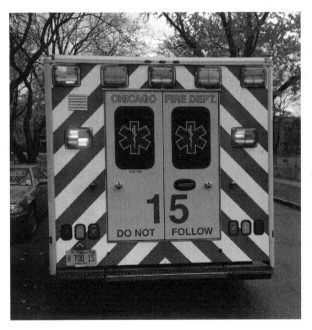

Chicago Fire Department Ambulance 15, a Chicago legend. Courtesy Paul Ciolino

When a thing, object, or city, obtains legendary status, it is usually for a very bad reason. The Hindenburg, Pearl Harbor, the Twin Towers,

United Flight 94---all bad, very bad, and not something with which one would want to be associated if you enjoy being on the right side of the lawn.

In the spirit of staying on the right side of the lawn, there is an "object" that is not only good, it is great. Chicago Fire Department Ambulance 15 might be the best piece of tires and metal that ever rolled down the very unforgiving streets of the west side of Chicago.

Many of the residents of Austin give very little thought to anything beyond their next buzz or felonious act. Ambulance Number 15 is a lone beacon of light and hope in a land that more resembles the blight and hopelessness of Port-a-Prince, Haiti than a modern world class city.

When you have been shot and are lying on North Cicero Avenue bleeding out, with twenty cops and a hundred twenty bystanders watching it happen, but doing nothing but watching, Ambulance 15 rolling up is *your* miracle. When you haven't taken your diabetes medication for three weeks, are in a diabetic seizure and absolutely no one around has a clue how to help, Ambulance 15 appears like a vision of Heaven.

When you are a lifelong asthmatic and you thought it was a good idea to shoot up a bag of heroin this morning, which triggered an attack that caused your lungs to shut down, and you are slowly, torturously, drowning from excess fluid in your lungs, Ambulance 15 comes rumbling up before you drop dead in the alley. Such are the moments that Ambulance 15 is both witness to and participant in the real world.

Ambulance 15 is the gold standard in the CFD's EMS armament. Its reputation is well deserved. Day to day, year in and year out, Ambulance 15 and its men and women may be the most consistent, largest piece of lifesaving equipment in the history of modern lifesaving equipment.

Anywhere from 18 to 30 times in a 24-hour period, Ambulance 15 rolls from one tragedy to the next. In between, cops, citizens and anyone who can whistle, wave their hands, or dive in front of it, are flagging it down. If Ambulance 15 was a horse, it would have to be shot every thirty days from overuse.

Lucky for most of us, the Jay DiGiovannis of the world don't spend a lot of time reading this data, nor does he spend much time considering these purported facts and figures.

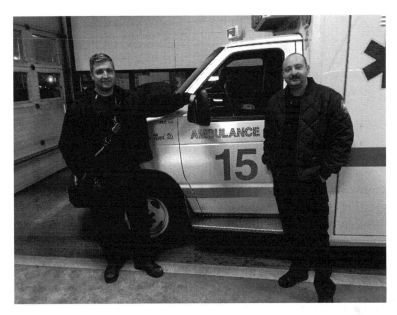

CFD Paramedic's Ambulance Commander Jay DiGiovanni,
and Mike Kuryla, November 2015. Paul Ciolino

Twenty-Four

The author's experience in ambulances has been limited to being a guest in them on occasion. Having never worked in one and then jumping into one of the busiest in the world is a little disconcerting. You can't help or offer advice. You are pretty much a ghost and the last thing you want to do is become a headline in tomorrow's paper. So, armed with a notebook and camera, with little fanfare, I climbed into the back of DiGiovani's office and for the next twenty-four hours witnessed a miracle.

Run Number One: It's 07:32 hrs on a blustery stormy windblown, November Veteran's Day and Mike Kuryla is manhandling his four-ton, rolling emergency room down Division and playing the lights, siren, and EMS computer, like a one-handed, idiot savant playing a grand concert piano. The original Apollo Astronauts didn't have to handle anything as convoluted and complicated as this, but Kuryla's fingers never stop. It seems every moron with access to a car is doing their level best to rear-end, T-bone, or have a head on collision with him and Ambulance 15.

Traffic laws are generally ignored and abandoned at the earliest opportunity. Kuryla handles the "bus" or "Ambo" like a NASCAR driver at Daytona. In and out, swerving around people who slam on their brakes for no obvious reason. He is non-plussed over the whole routine. For the next 24 hours, this is his own private version of purgatory. He has long abandoned any hope of rhyme or reason. He just drives and dodges the four-ton behemoth, while at all times manipulating and twirling those knobs and gadgets.

Kuryla doesn't swear, scream or gesture. He calmly steers #15 around traffic, small bomb crater sized potholes, and pedestrians who think lights and sirens are synonymous with walking in front of ambulances and other emergency equipment whipping around the city. He doesn't drive fast or appear in any real hurry. As 15 glides up to a residence on Division Street, the well-rehearsed symphony of saving yet another life begins. He and his boss, Ambulance Commander Jay DiGiovanni, begin their waltz.

There is no conversation and no wasted or hurried movements. They have performed this dance thousands of times. They could do it blindfolded. They have done it with bullets flying around them like angry pissed off wasps. They are unfazed by all the drama swirling around them. They silently review every SOP, medical procedure and safety issue they may encounter. There is no 'Plan B' or alternative action considered. This is as real as it gets and they both understand the consequences. One wrong move, one tiny mental lapse, and someone dies or their life changes forever.

It's strangely quiet and for a minute or two, almost normal. There are not a lot of people milling about. All the drapes are drawn and no one peeks or rubbernecks. The neighbors are silent. DiGiovanni and Kuryla look bored. They appear passive, but nothing could be further from the truth. Watching the police respond to a home in Austin and then watching fire department personnel respond are two entirely different animals.

The Chicago Police officers are generally young guys. They are in shape and they don't so much walk or do anything in a casual manner. They play offense. They move with a purpose and you do not want to test their mood or resolve. Like Iraq and Afghanistan, as well as here in Austin, there is no second place. There are no debates. If you want to test them, nothing good will happen to you. In addition to going to jail, you will get your ass beat if you resist. Put a hand on them, or get stupid in any manner and very bad things will happen to you. This is a very subjective area and you don't get a vote. You respond immediately and without hesitation to direction, or suffer the consequences.

The Ambo guys are not the police. No guns, no bulletproof vests, and no backup unless they really need it. They are out there without a raft. They have no mechanical means of defending themselves. The community understands the difference. Well, they understand it as long as heroin, K-2, Weed, or PCP is not in the mix. Then all bets are off. About every third run will involve those drugs or alcohol or a combination of that and anything else that may be available, including cheap mouthwash.

For CFD personnel, the great equalizer on the street is "the look". It's difficult to explain, but like leadership, you know it when you see it. The "look" is in lieu of "the gun" as in "I am the police and I will shoot you".

But firemen are forbidden from carrying any kind of offensive weapon, so they are forced to pull out '*The Look*' when things start to go south. '*The Look*,' properly utilized, translated means, "Look pal, I don't have 'The Gun' and I can't shoot you, but if you keep dicking around with my boys or me, I will toss your narrow ass off the roof." Based on statistical data, '*The Look*' just may be the ticket when dealing with the disingenuous in Austin. It is only to be employed on real dickweeds. Part of the warrior code and all that.

The call came over as "*a male having trouble breathing*". DiGiovanni said, "Probably drugs." They pull up in front of a fairly nice-looking home and the ritual begins. Two-inch thick Ambo doors slam like oversized bank vaults and Kuryla walks over to the passenger side to remove a "chair stretcher" from a side compartment. DiGiovanni opens the side door and deposits his Panasonic "Toughbook" (a military grade portable computer) on a shelf. The computer is DiGiovanni's go-to for everything---drugs, treatment, actions taken, patient data, etc. It is blazing fast and never more than a few steps from Jay's reach. The "Toughbook" is unusual in that it is simply and amazingly fast. Data input is simple and teetering on real "Artificial Intelligence".

There is a fire truck present upon their arrival and three uniformed firemen are already in the house. (The fire trucks often respond independently if they think the paramedics are jammed up or running late.) Often they are dispatched if the Ambos are all tied up. There are generally enough trained personnel with medical equipment to deal with the big issues. If DiGiovanni is *The Duke*, these guys are the royal family.

As soon as DiGiovanni arrives, he is in charge. Everyone backs up half a step and Jay assumes control of the scene. No one speaks unless Jay asks him or her a direct question. As an ambulance commander, he is of equal rank with a captain. He is responsible for any and all medical decisions. He, and everyone there, knows and understands this by regulation, as well as intuitively.

There is a very interesting dynamic afoot here and few civilians would ever understand it. They would not recognize it and most would not care to understand what is happening. It's very subtle, even magical, in its simplicity and movement. None of the firemen openly recognize or act subservient in any manner. This is the last rodeo. It is old school and without question the last non-sports team environment where men still very much act like men.

No one cares about your rank or time on the job. What counts here, what really matters is performance. Can you cut it? Are you there for your brothers? When the shit hits the fan do you run into the line of fire or do you start looking for an excuse to do something out of the line of fire? Fat, skinny, old, young, muscled up and cut, dumpy with a beer belly, or last day before retirement---none of that means squat to these guys.

"Are you a wolf or a lamb?" That is the question and every fiber of their being screams this. The brotherhood demands it and God help anyone who thinks they are going to change it. If you are going to play on this team that is the core standard. Man, woman, white, or minority, you are welcomed into the brotherhood as long as you can abide by this. Not everyone is meant to do this and the weeding out of those who thought they could "slick their way" into the brotherhood is uncompromising and resolute. You will not be long for a working west side firehouse or ambulance.

The fire department attempts to impose its will on the troops. Hair and mustache regulations, uniforms, shoes, boots, and a hundred other rules, are enforced in general. No one gets too out of control.

But there is a lot of individuality leaking out all over the floor. It's minor and not worth getting into a pissing contest or a disciplinary issue bubbling up, but it's there in a dozen little different ways the men push that envelope. The brotherhood resists its masters at every opportunity, but only to a point. The general consensus is, "Will my men run into that burning building and save a stranger's life?" On the West Side, the answer is without a doubt, "Yes". They will sacrifice themselves without thought or hesitation. That is what separates these amazing and giving men and women from the rest of us. It is mystic in its simplicity.

Once DiGiovanni and Kuryla assume control, the responding firemen, decked out in duty pants, the ever cool fire department T-shirt, and manly-man suspenders holding it all up, take a step back. They are bit players at this point, but the cool factor is still present. The more fire-scarred and nastier the ensemble, the cooler the look. The old-timers' T-shirts are all pretty standard. They look like your dad dressed up as a big city badass fireman.

The younger guys, well that is where this gets a little dicey. They wear a medley of old and new. Old enough to look salty, and new high tech stuff that is hip. Their T-shirts are cut high and tight, better to show off those badass guns. Chicks dig big guns, especially tatted up big guns. "Shit, I'm flying that flag, regulations be damned."

The young dudes sport so many tattoos you think the Hell's Angels just showed up at your house. Sleeve tattoos (basically cover one's entire arm) are well represented. Neck tattoos, formerly reserved for gangsters and prison inmates, are now common. In the firehouse, the boys display enough ink on every other part of their body to make one think they are on a Navy Destroyer rather than the west side of Chicago.

These younger firemen are different---more muscular, spikey haircuts, health freaks, watch their diet---these guys are definitely new wave. Their gym (which the firemen pay for and stock) would make most professional sports team gyms look like a Mario Tricoci day spa. The motif is more torture chamber cool then workout space. The older guys seem indifferent. They mastered cool in the 80's. "Hey junior, jump on that roof and grab the family hamster." "No problem boss." The hamster gets retrieved as if it's an infant. No, the old guys are way more conservative, but the new breed of warrior is still a warrior.

The old timers don't know tattoo from Ragu. They believe their job is simple. Guard the eternal flame. Protect a century plus of tradition, bravery, honor, and loyalty. Do not dishonor the service. Bring every man home, do your job in a professional manner, fight and die for "The Brotherhood". If you do, then it's all good. Every generation has their doubts about the next. It's the natural order of things. In the firehouse, this is really amplified. Maintaining the status and honor of "The Brotherhood" is the mission. All good things flow from within its confines. It is the mother lode that will continue giving as long as it is honored.

Jay is in full paramedic mode immediately. There is no wasted motion, no unnecessary movement or conversation. He assesses and watches. He hits the patient with a litany of questions right away, without drama or raising his voice. "Where's it hurt? Do you know where you are? What day is it? We're going to take you out to the ambulance and help you out, OK?" If it will get dicey, this is usually when it happens.

Mike isn't saying much. He's unfolding the stretcher chair. He's arranging the straps. He's watching and waiting for it to turn. He explains later. "They go from passive to full fight mode in 0-60. You have to strap them in fast. Don't give them time to debate or think. Get control, watch the bystanders. Above all else don't let anyone get nuts on you." He's dead serious and he looks like it. He's polite, professional, but there is a feeling of simmering violence right below the surface. He has mastered *The Look*. Mike does not play. If he doesn't go home tomorrow morning, it will not be because he wasn't paying attention.

They get the guy in the ambulance, on the stretcher and strapped down tight. Mike is at the bottom. He's checking blood pressure. It's high. He checks his sugar to rule out diabetic issues. It's 164, not horrible, but a little elevated. He ties a rubber strap around the patient's upper arm to help pump up his veins, pulls an IV needle out and wipes down the back of the man's hand. He slips the needle in with practiced ease. The patient, not happy, starts to squirm. He knows what's coming.

Jay works the top end. He whips out a pen light, checks both eyes of the patient and says "Sir, how much heroin did you do today?" The guy is silent for a moment, then says, "I did a couple bags this morning". Jay says, "Ok sir, we're going to give you some medicine to make you feel better". Jay pulls out some liquid Naloxone,[20] hands it to Mike who inserts it into the IV. The effect is almost immediate as the patient starts to sweat, looks around, and is more alert. He quits struggling against the stretcher straps. He has a look of defeat on his face, but he's agitated. He states, "I don't feel good". Jay says "Sir, you'll feel better in a little while".

Mike gets out of the back of the ambulance and they are off to the nearest emergency room, which is West Suburban Hospital in Oak Park, Illinois. In less than five minutes, the patient is wheeled in. Jay and Mike stop at the first desk in the emergency room and Jay briefs the admitting nurse in a machine gun like speech full of medical jargon. If you were not a trained professional and versed in the language of medicine, you would think Jay was speaking in tongues. It comes fast and furious---almost sounds like Star Trek's Captain Kirk speaking Klingon.

The admitting nurse simply says, "Room Three". Mike and Jay wheel the patient down to Room Three with a platoon of ER nurses trailing behind. They transfer the patient to a hospital stretcher and the nurses take over. Jay wishes the man well and grabs the ever-present Panasonic laptop that is always under the patient's head under the top half of the ambo stretcher. He goes into an office that the paramedics use to write up the never-ending paperwork. Mike strips the ambulance stretcher sheets and gets fresh ones, then returns to the ambulance where he cleans and sanitizes the business end of it. In nineteen runs, in the next 24 hours, this procedure will not vary.

While typing and printing his reports, Jay explains the run. "He was having trouble breathing because he was obese, out of shape and older than his years. Add heroin to the mix and he is a walking health disaster. The problem is that the dope changes everything. We hit them with a small dose of the Narcan and it usually brings them around. You have to be careful with it because, one, it pisses them off; two, it immediately ruins their buzz, and three, they had it before and they don't like it. It makes them dope sick and they usually have no idea how bad in shape they were in when we got there. It's a tricky moment because you don't want to hit them with too much and make them more sick and even more combative."

When asked how he knew it was heroin, Jay replies, "As soon as you put the light on their eyes and the pupils look like pinholes, you know it. They don't react to the light and they look smaller then the tip of a fine pen. Opiates do that and heroin is the opiate of choice in Austin."

It's a slow start of the day. Seldom does Ambulance 15 get back to the firehouse before the end of shift. As soon as they finish one call, another comes in within minutes. The paramedics work twenty-four hours on and then are off for the next three days.

The firemen on the ladder and engineer trucks work twenty-four on as well, but they only get the next two days off. At one time, firemen were not happy about this arrangement. Not at the Chicago Avenue firehouse. They have a front row seat to the madness. They watch the paramedics on Ambulance15 killing themselves daily. There are generally no breaks in the action. The paramedics usually don't have time to eat. They have to steal five minutes to go the bathroom. The pressure is relentless and it seldom varies. The firemen on Chicago Avenue get it. They watch over their paramedics. They always save plates of food for them. They are very conscious of the fact that DiGiovanni and Kuryla are slowly, but certainly, killing themselves out there.

Run Number Two: 11:18 hrs. Jay and Mike fast walk towards Ambulance 15. They have a call of *"Unknown cause"*. Jay explains this can mean anything. We will not have a clue until we get there. They arrive at West End and Chicago Ave. The loss of beauty of the homes in this part of Austin is depressing. Long ago, these were magnificent, stately homes. In other more affluent parts of the city, these homes would fetch up to a million dollars or more. Here in Austin, they are almost giving them away. Most of them have been split up into small apartment buildings. Zoning laws are non-existent in Austin.

Two young kids on the corner selling drugs don't miss a beat as the Ambo rolls by them. Although they can't be more then thirteen or fourteen years old, they already have that territorial predator look. They are "eye fucking" Ambulance 15 as it rolls by. Mike gives them "The (CFD) Look" right back. It's a draw. They stay on the corner and Mike pulls up in the front of the building where the 911 call originated.

The patient's adult daughter meets them on the first floor. She explains that her mother has an appointment with her doctor. Dragging the stretcher chair up a long flight of stairs, they meet with the woman. Entering the apartment is like walking into a used medical equipment sales room. Laying everywhere are wheel chairs, canes, three-pronged walking sticks, and crutches. The woman sits in the dining room. She is enormous. She is, for certain, not anorexic or bulimic.

She explains that she just needs help getting down the stairs and into her car for an appointment with her physician. She isn't sick and she does not require any emergency medical attention. Jay and Mike are courteous and professional. They treat her like a VIP. Their tone is respectful and accommodating. They load her into the stretcher chair, strap her in, and start the dangerous downward descent.

Maneuvering through hallways and doorways that were not designed to code for the Americans with Disabilities Act, Jay and Mike push, pull, carry and sweat their way down the rickety stairs and crumbling concrete porch to the sidewalk. One of the patient's daughters stands by a Mercedes Benz SUV. Jay and Mike assist the woman out of the chair and into the Mercedes. The woman is treated like American royalty. Jay and Mike look like they just did a Pilates class with Mia Hamm.

No one complains over the obvious misuse of the 911 system. In Austin, the Ambo is almost like calling Uber. If you call and can get around the screening process, the Ambo will come. Never mind that you kept a million dollars of equipment and two highly trained and competent paramedics tied up for twenty minutes. It's all about you.

The boys are not upset in the least. They get a lot of these calls. They feel their duty is to the community. They put a Bandaid® on every wound they come across. If it requires a strong back and a little sweat, they are glad to help. This is *their* reality. They have neither the time nor patience to lecture anyone. The CFD model is *"We're Here When You Need Us"*. Ambulance 15 turns no soul away. They seem to be everywhere.

Later, Jay explains it this way, "We get a lot of these type calls. Certainly it abuses a too spread out department. But we go. We don't judge and we don't refuse anyone service. That woman that we loaded into the car needed us. It was somewhat of a bullshit call and they knew it. I didn't feel a need to rub it in. it's likely we'll do it again".

Run Number Three: 11:35 hrs. Ambulance 15 is dispatched on an abdominal distress call. The opera starts the same way every time. Up the stairs they go. It seems no one ever gets sick on the first floor. They enter a small two-bedroom apartment.

In the tiny living room there is an ancient looking TV blasting 'Sponge Bob'. Two little kids sit there, hypnotized. They pay zero attention to the paramedics and their medical equipment. With the kids, sitting on the couch watching the cartoon, is an adult man. Not a sound or word of acknowledgement.

In a small bedroom off the living room, the patient is wrapped in every blanket and towel she could get her hands on. She is the size of a skinny ten-year-old. The patient and room have the look and feel of Somalia, not Chicago. On a good day, she might weigh 90 pounds. With her sunken eyes, she looks like a refugee camp survivor. She is clearly in pain and great discomfort. DiGiovanni keeps the questions to a minimum. Mike and Jay wrap her up and put her in the stretcher. They're in and out in about four minutes.

As she is wheeled out, 'Sponge Bob' plays on. Nobody says anything. The kids ignore her. The boyfriend doesn't even bother to look up. They get her on the Ambo stretcher and they go into serious, high paramedic gear---BP, sugar, temp, close inspection for injuries. Jay hits her with a dozen rapid-fire questions. "Are you pregnant? When was your last period? Your last meal, what did you eat?" He circles and narrows down the causes. Mike drops an IV bag and works the systems. The woman is getting the princess treatment and looks happy that someone is finally paying attention to her. The guys speak softly and respectfully. They always ask permission to do the tiniest things. *The Duke* is all business. This is clearly a very ill woman-child and the air is charged with pending disaster.

Giovanni's tone is never excited. He speaks to every patient the same way. He is at the height of his considerable powers and people just intuitively understand that *The Duke* is there to help. He is the P. Diddy of Austin, the ultimate cool dude. The patients respond in spite of their mistrust of any uniformed government agent.

Jay is oblivious to all of this. He works the problem. He is analytical and focused. He lives in fear of blowing one. It is what keeps him up and the adrenalin quietly surging for almost every moment of his twenty-four-hour shift.

There is a symmetry and purpose to every movement. The medicine, the technology, the paramedics all work in one fluid motion. When it works, it's magical. It is lifesaving and it's poetic. The patients are generally clueless to what's going on around them. They are sick and in pain. Observing all this, understanding what's going on and what the end result will be, is about as much fun as you can have with your clothes on. It's still early and *The Duke* is rocking it tonight.

The patient gets the full Monty. No stone left unturned. She has won the paramedic lottery today and, through the mask of pain, she understands this. They transport her to Norwegian American Hospital. Jay goes into the high-speed explanation. The patient watches with a child-like wonder. She is stable and looking a little less stressed.

The triage nurse tells Mike and Jay to put the patient in a chair in the public waiting room. It's high noon and the ER is rocking. There is no bed immediately available. A security person gets her situated for a long wait. *The Duke* is not happy. He does not like to see people treated like livestock. In this case, he will have to live with it.

Run Number Four: 11:55 hrs: It was his 18th birthday yesterday when the party started. He was still going strong when he passed out on his mother's kitchen floor. Upon arrival there is a fire truck and crew present. Two firemen are coming down the steps with the birthday boy between them. He is a skinny, typical 18-year-old who has not yet filled out. His eyes are closed. He is mumbling, head bobbing like an old doll. The firemen dump him into the back of the ambulance. His mom and an older sister trail behind. They are pissed at junior and Mom wants to "beat his ass." She's both embarrassed and ticked.

Jay and Mike get into the routine. The kid is carping and bitching non-stop. No one is paying attention to what he wants. A conversation with Mom reveals the kid has been smoking K-2, a manmade designer drug that can be purchased on the Internet.[21] If you think for one second that this stuff is harmless, think again. It is both dangerous and unpredictable. Exhibit One is lying on the stretcher, headed to the hospital. Maybe Nancy Reagan was right.

Run Number Five/12:08 hrs: The 911 dispatchers always sound the same. Bored, indifferent, and even casual. They don't have the cool, Chuck Yeager country gentleman pilot voice announcing disasters like reading a letter from Mom, but they have an urban big city, cool vibe sound that comes out bored and indifferent. This is 15's twenty-four-seven soundtrack.

They pull up on West Lotus and there is a fire truck present. The crew is upstairs when 15 arrives on scene. It's a chest pain call so everyone will hustle on this one because a heart attack will, unequivocally, kill you. It is quickly determined that the chest pains are caused by smoking dope. The thirty-something female is loaded in the Ambo. Her BP is high, EKG[22] normal. Jay gives her some baby aspirin and nitroglycerin. She starts feeling better and they take her West Suburban ER. Like everyone else, she is treated with every possible courtesy. *The Duke* is thoughtful and reassures her with every movement. In her own personal fog, she does appear grateful.

Run Number Six/13:16 hrs: Another fire truck crew is on scene when 15 arrives out of their area on North Avenue. Di Giovanni assumes control. The victim is in his late 50's and clearly in pain. His son and daughter-in-law look worried. Kuryla loads him in the chair and the firemen carry him down the crumbling, concrete stairs.

The patient gets loaded and Jay and Mike move fast. The man is very uncomfortable. He looks sick and miserable. BP is very high, sugar is high. What problem does this guy not have? At least his EKG is normal. The guy screams when Mike finally finds a suitable vein. He did not like the IV needle.

Jay questions the victim *in Spanish*. The meds start kicking in and it's off to West Suburban again. Jay's fairly certain that the man has an obstructed bowel. No apparent street drugs involved. The man is admitted and passed off to the ER Doc. DiGiovanni does the paperwork. 15 is in service before they leave the ER. Who needs an interpreter? Not *The Duke*.

Run Number Seven/14:05 hrs: *"Man down in a gas station."* Upon 15's arrival, they walk into the gas station/mini mart. It's busy and hectic. From behind two inches of bulletproof glass, the gas station owners point as the paramedics walk in. Lying in front of a cooler on his side is a man, barely coherent. He starts to rise, but he's very wobbly. He is also pissed off. He was taking a nap and he makes it very clear he does not want an ambulance. The store is crowded. People step over and around him. No one wants to participate in this drama. On the 'pissed off and I'm going to fight' scale of one to ten, he is a five and rising quickly. With the help of a friend who has walked in, he reluctantly climbs and falls into the back of 15 after a whole lot of swearing and threats.

The fight scale continues to rise. Kuryla is watching carefully. He's not saying much but his body language is all business. Jay's rap is not having much affect. The nap dude is 'motherfucking' and daring everyone within earshot. He clearly wants to fight. The napper is 60 years old and lean and mean. A life of living in the streets has aged him considerably. Toss in some dope and his is more like a can of five-gallon gasoline than a human being.

DiGiovanni is tiring of being 'Jay the nice concerned health professional'. He abandons that strategy and turns into 'Ambulance Commander DiGiovanni'. There is little compassion in his voice as he lays it out for Nap Man. "Sir, you are going to the hospital. You are sick or impaired and you clearly require some help. I am the only person here who makes that decision. You want to be a little nicer, or do we restrain you?"

Through the fog of whatever drug Nap Man partied with today, he seems to recognize the non-negotiation tone in Jay's voice. He's still talking shit, but he is clearly defeated. He will reluctantly cooperate.

Kuryla looks a little disappointed. He has not yet worked out today and he thought Nap Man might be a nice warm-up. Nap Man is delivered to Loreto Hospital on Central Ave. The ER department nurses look none too happy with this patient. Jay calls in "Back in service" before he hits the back door.

There is a break in the action. The weather is turning quick. The none too friendly Chicago winter starts to raise its ugly head and dampens the street action. Jay and Mike return to the firehouse and begin minor maintenance on 15. The work is never done. The boys are in constant and steady motion as they get 15 ready for action, then proceed to the firehouse kitchen eating area.

They load up on fresh coffee and a variety of cookies, snacks, and fruit. The firemen clearly love these two. There is a profound unspoken reverence towards these two paramedics on every level. They throw every creature comfort at them every time they return to the house. Mark Kovacevich, a younger fireman and 82nd Airborne Veteran, is in a state of constant movement and chatter. "Want some cookies, chocolate cake, bananas?" The diet at Chicago Avenue is a fifteen-year-old hormonal boy's wet dream. The food smells as good as it tastes. Eating here, you could turn into a fat ass really quick. However, there are no chubby guys here. They burn it off as fast as they inhale it.

Run Number Eight/16:54 hrs: It's full dark outside and rain is coming down sideways. 911 blasts an *"injured person in a parking lot"* call. Fifteen rolls slowly, but steadily, towards the latest drama act in Austin. They arrive and find a woman of gigantic girth sitting in the backseat of her son's car in the grocery store parking lot. Kuryla diagnoses this one before he grabs the stretcher chair. "Probably a slip and fall lawsuit case. She needs to get to the ER to solidify her claim."

The woman immediately starts to yell about her back. "I can't move. The pain is terrible." Jay and Mike ease her out of the back seat onto the stretcher chair. She appears to come out of the car in sections. Her son stands by silently. He is in a hurry to bail out of there. He looks on, very bored. The car is in gear and moving before she gets strapped to the stretcher. He doesn't ask where 15 is taking her.

In spite of what he might be thinking, as the fat lady sings loudly, *The Duke* treats her like Princess Diana. It's not fake or disingenuous. The woman calms down and becomes quieter and friendlier. They roll into West Suburban. The ER is jammed. Jay runs through a very brief summary. The triage nurse doesn't even look up. "Put her out front in the public waiting room." Jay and Mike wordlessly wheel her out of the ER and into the waiting room. A bored security guard reluctantly gets up and retrieves a king-sized wheelchair. The opera ends with Jay saying, "Good luck to y'all, Ma'am". She grins a little and looks at the security guard. "What y'all got to eat?" Fifteen departs and yet another happy customer settles in for a long night.

Run Number Nine/17:31 hrs: A 76-year-old lady is in severe abdominal distress on West Washington. Upon arrival, Jay and Mike maneuver around filthy mattresses on the floor, three little kids, and an apartment full of roaches. Mike whispers, "Don't lean on anything or sit down, you'll get covered in bugs". Great advice. The patient is sick, really sick. Pain oozes from every pore. Her daughter tells Jay, "She can't eat and she can't go to the bathroom". A lifetime of bad food, diet, and lack of exercise is coming home to roost.

She gets wrapped and transported quick. There is no fooling around. The questions come from Jay in a rapid-fire technique. He is calm and purposeful. He and Mike hustle. They both look worried, but in complete control. All kinds of medicine and needles are deployed. The vital signs are all shaky. Jay works the radio at the same time. He tells an unseen emergency room doctor what he's dealing with. It's Klingon time again. The doc says, "Transport as soon as possible."

Mike wheels 15 into the West Suburban Sally Port with the ease of Dale Earnhardt rolling into a pit stop. They roll her in and three nurses trail them carrying "nurse stuff". She is transferred to an ER stretcher and the paperwork and clean up start. Jay types up his report and radios in their "in service status". When asked why he doesn't take a break or ease up for ten minutes, Jay responds thoughtfully. "Our district is constantly going. There is not much down time. I never want anyone to catch a call, especially a bad one, because I decided we need a break. You don't do that on the West Side. We don't do that to each other. We are a team and we take care of each other no matter how inconvenient, or how tired we might be. You don't want to be 'that guy'. It's just that simple."

The Duke doesn't mess around. It's all business, all the time. Life pretty much sucks on the West Side, but once every fourth day the sun does shine on the old dog's ass because *The Duke* is in the house.

Run Number Ten/18:45hrs: "The Wildman"[23] is not having a good day. He is curled up in front of his apartment door in a fetal position with a plastic shopping bag full of pharmaceutical prescription drugs. A concerned neighbor stands by. You know the patient's name is "Wildman" because its boldly tattooed on his neck. He didn't quite make it inside. He is 45-years-old. A lifetime of hard drugs and Type One Diabetes has taken a toll. "Wildman" is barely coherent and in bad shape. His arms are covered in tattoos, mostly religious symbols and crosses. Not a bad looking guy, he does the heroin nod while Jay tried to get him upright. It's a losing battle.

He gets strapped in the chair stretcher and down the stairs he goes. They navigate to the bottom and "Wildman" remembers his pills. Jay grabs the house keys, bounces up the stairs, grabs the bag, places it inside the door, double locks the door and comes back down. *The Duke*---he is full service all the time.

"Wildman" gets transferred, strapped in, and hit with the Narcan. Predictably, the Narcan does its magic. The "Wildman" is sick and informs Jay that he has Pancreatitis,[24] in addition to his other problems. His blood sugar is through the roof. Jay and Mike give him the full Monty and he comes around. "Wildman" gets it. He is respectful and appreciative. He is wheeled into West Suburban ER and the nurses go into their act.

Run Number Eleven/20:50 hrs: "Don Giovanni,"[25] perhaps Mozart's greatest opera, was written around 1787. John "Jay" DiGiovanni, (*The Duke*) was born in the southern suburbs of Chicago around 1970. The comparison is weak, but the greatness is similar. Mozart was not known for saving lives, but he wrote great operas. *The Duke* doesn't write great operas, but he is a lifesaving machine.

"Unknown problem" on West Division Street. #15 rolls up on a guy repeatedly falling off his bicycle onto the wet parking lot of a convenience store. The bike is brand new and expensive. The man's uncle is there and he called 911. He is pissed and he's tired of arguing with his adult nephew who is clearly lit up. He informs the paramedics "that asshole is drunk and high on heroin". The nephew says, "I only had a few beers and a small bag of heroin." That fine distinction is not lost on the paramedics. The uncle however, is done and out of there.

Paramedic Mike Kuryla solves the problem. Heroin/Beer guy and bike make it to West Suburban in one piece.

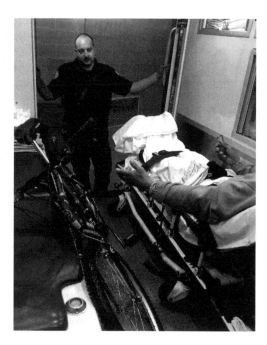

CFD Mike Kuryla negotiates with a patient. November 2015. Paul Ciolino

The standing-up, falling down patient progresses slowly towards the back of #15, assisted by the boys. This guy is going to the hospital upright or parallel. Mike does not much care which way. The big question is, what happens to the bike? This is clearly not a problem for #15. They are not the bicycle police and they have enough problems with "Heroin/Beer Guy. CFD's business model does not address these lofty issues.

The boys do not disappoint. After a discussion worthy of CNN's 'Crossfire', Mike solves the problem. The bike and "Heroin/Beer Guy" get the million-dollar ride to West Suburban. The patient gets hit with Narcan and the bike drip-dries next to him in the back of #15. The bike looks a little less dope sick than "Heroin/Beer Guy". Everyone gets wheeled into the ER---the bike right along with its owner. The ER nurse calls for a security guy who takes the bike out and puts it on the secured dock with a bunch of other nice bikes. Who knew?

Run Number Twelve/21:35 hrs: It's an illegal basement apartment meant to be only a basement on North Laramie. These houses are all pre-1920 and they look and smell like it. A 63-year-old heavyset guy sits on the edge of his bed, holding his right arm and clearly in excruciating pain. He's dressed in a clean, white T-shirt and nice jeans. His bed and room are spotless. A very old TV sits on a TV tray that is about to collapse. This is "Divorced Dad/Spartan" living at life's simplest.

The first thing the man says when the boys hit the front door and walk into a room, turning lights on along the way is, "I'm sorry to bother you guys." Jay looks like he won the lotto. Holy Christ, a patient without a drug issue mucking up the medical problem(s). Jay's body temp may have risen a degree in quiet celebration. He bounds over to the man and says, "Sir, it's no bother at all. We're here to help you." The guy is so relieved he looks like he is ready to cry. Jay talks to him and treats him like it's his own father, rather than a stranger.

It's the first time in fourteen and a half hours that anyone has come close to appearing grateful. The man is almost embarrassed for calling for the much-needed help. There is no wasted motion getting him into the back of 15. The ladder guys show up and are there to help. They walk in and give the place "The Look" just in case there is someone lurking about. The ladder guys manage the bad ass/really cool fireman look without an audience. Like the Boy Scouts, they are always prepared. They help load the patient and secure the apartment. Who needs Brinks when the CFD is around?

The pain is nine on a one to ten scale. DiGiovanni is in full tilt medical problem solving mode. Mike quietly, but constantly, reassures the man. They are humming. The buzz in 15 is palpable. They wheel him into West Suburban. The welcoming committee is in full force. Jay and Mike start the closing out process. Jay says, "You have to be very careful. With a lot of these patients, the drugs mask the real problems. You have to be very diligent because they can code in a second.

You have to be ready to jump on it. You gotta dig deep. This guy had me worried. He had some serious health issues. He looked really bad for a few minutes. I'm glad he called us."

Jay is reflective. He thinks the man may have had an aorta[26] issue. It could have been caused by a half dozen different problems. It could very well kill him. Jay will continue to check up on him throughout the night. These are the cases that keep *The Duke* fretting all night.

Run Number Thirteen/22:13 hrs: "*15, sick person on Cicero Avenue*" Off they go to a vague call and an even more vague address. 15 cruises North Cicero Avenue looking for the sick guy. It's raining like a cow pissing on a flat rock and visibility is about four and a half feet. Finally, after about ten minutes of searching, Mike spots a young guy in his rear view mirror waving at them. He backs the bus up a good hundred meters, thinking this must be the "sick person's friend" coming to guide us to him. Not a chance. The thirty-something-year-old picture of health fairly leaps into the side door of 15.

Hero Guy: "Sorry to call you guys, but I wasn't feeling too good."

Jay: "What's the problem, sir?"

Hero Guy: "Well, where do I start? My wife and me just had a baby. I haven't really slept in a week. I drink thirty cups of coffee a day and I started work at seven this morning and I haven't eaten anything except (holding up a bag of chips) these Cheetos. Oh yeah, and I bought a house and moved to Lisle (a suburb of Chicago). My truck is running like shit and while I'm welding I breathe in all these cancer-causing chemicals and I smoke way too much."

Jay: "Do you want to go to the hospital?"

Hero Guy: "Not really. I can't afford it. Can you just check me out? Make sure I'm not having a heart attack?"

Jay: "That's what we're here for. Let's take a look at you."

Meanwhile, "Hero Guy" pounds Cheetos like it's the Last Supper. Jay checks his BP, sugar, etc. "Hero Guy" is not so much crazy, but maybe in need of a marginally competent dietitian as opposed to an ambulance.

Jay: "Sir, your BP is a little high, otherwise you're looking pretty good. Maybe you should dial back the cigarettes and caffeine?"

Hero Guy: "Well, maybe it's the three super-sized Red Bulls I pound every day."

Jay: "Sir, that may make you feel a little anxious, as well."

Hero Guy: "Phew! I'm feeling better now. Man, I love you guys. You are heroes. When I used to drive a cab twenty-two hours a day, seven days a week, I was a hero like youse guys."

Mike perks up with the hero comment, but not enough to ask him to clarify the hero stuff. His participation proves to be unnecessary.

Jay: "Um huh."

Hero Guy: "No shit. I saved a lady's life as she was about to be raped by another cab driver. I had a young lady fare and we drove by this cab and a woman was fighting with a cab driver. She was standing outside the cab hitting the dude through his window. The dude was hanging on to her jacket sleeve. Anyways we drove by and I say to my fare, 'You think we should go back and help? My fare goes 'No, I'm tired. Just get me home.'"

Jay: "Sir, do you want to go to the hospital now?"

Hero Guy: "No, no, wait I gotta finish this. So I say the hell with my fare and I bang a U-turn and go back. Here's the hero part. I get the lady in my cab and I take her home. I don't charge her. That makes me a hero like youse guys right?"

Jay: "It certainly does, Sir. We can still take you to a hospital, if you want."

Hero Guy: "Nah, I'm feeling pretty good now. Think I'll go get my truck and go home. I hope my wife ain't pissed."

The Cheetos are almost all gone now. Kuryla, whose fingers are drumming on a shelf in a Ginger Baker like tempo looks like he is ready to strangle "Hero Guy."

Jay: "Sir, it's been a pleasure. Call anytime."

"Hero Guy" leaps off the back of 15 and trots off into the night. There will not be a lot of paper on this one.

Run Number Fourteen/23:33 hrs: "Angry Granny" is not happy. Sitting on the floor of her living room, wrapped up in a filthy comforter, "Angry Granny", all of 91 years and maybe a hundred pounds of her is pissed. She is not happy and the boys get an earful. "Fuck all of you. I ain't leaving and you can't make me leave." Her adult son cowers behind a wall in the darkened living room. He is old and not looking all that great himself. He wants her gone. It's obvious that he is pretty willing to do or say anything to get "Angry Granny" out of here.

The single family home has seen much better days. "Angry Granny" has lived there since the 60's. The rug she sits on is covered in fecal matter. It smells like urine, as does the comforter the boys are trying to untangle "Angry Granny" from. She is not cooperating and this is one time where muscle is useless. "Angry Granny" is not going without a fight.

She is confused and dazed. She is probably dehydrated. Dementia has clearly set in. She wants the paramedics to call her mother. Angry Granny's mother died in 1990. "Angry Granny" says, "I don't give a shit. You call my Momma right fucking now you bastards." Mike and Jay look as if they are waiting for the big Exorcist money shot where the head starts spinning and green bile pours out of the mouth like a wall of green poison. The language does not match up with the tiny, frail, old woman who not too long ago, in all likelihood, was a woman who would rather choke than curse.

Finally, "Angry Granny" gets loaded and strapped down. This does not improve her mood. However, her middle-aged son looks almost giddy when she finally leaves for West Suburban. Mike tells him where they are taking his mother. He mumbles something about going there. Nobody believes him. He is done with this and perhaps in the back of his mind he realizes his turn in the back of 15 may be coming sooner rather than later.

"Angry Granny" is admitted, but the nurses don't fare much better than the boys. They, too, get the "Angry Granny" treatment. "Angry Granny" does not discriminate. Everybody gets a "fuck you" tonight.

Jay starts the paperwork. There is not much to it. He looks up a number and calls a hotline for the Illinois Department of Aging. He gets a young woman on the line. The conversation is unnecessarily long. The call-taker insists the woman must have been abused. Jay tries to explain that he saw no signs of abuse. The woman and her son need help, not cops. Finally, after about a half hour, he gets through to her. The call ends and Jay puts 15 back into the rotation. There will be little rest for the "Angry Granny" jabbers tonight.

Run Number Fifteen/01:25 hrs: Any run after "Angry Granny" is cake. Kuryla would rather roll up to a gunfight in the middle of Cicero Avenue than deal with "Angry Granny" again. He gets his wish. 15 is rolling on, *"See a man who has been poisoned"* call. Even *The Duke*, whose patience knows no limits, looks a little relieved. Yet another vague address on Cicero Avenue, but this time no detective work is needed. There are seven uniformed and plainclothes police officers milling about the poison "victim". The cops are dressed for serious business. In Austin, there is no such thing as casual. They appear to be dressed for action in Iraq or Afghanistan, not in a Chicago neighborhood. Some of them, no doubt, have spent time in those places. Their whole demeanor and body language suggest anything but "Officer Friendly". No, in Austin policing is serious business. These guys don't write traffic tickets. They don't do routine patrol. They don't do bicycle thefts. They do "guns & dope". They do shootings, shots fired and they do 10-1, (officer needs immediate assistance).

The "poison victim" is upright and coherent. He is a little edgy and has a little bit of an attitude, but he has calculated the odds and decided he had better behave himself. The boys extract him from the bevy of cops and get him into the bus. He slowly reverts back to tough guy status and is a little belligerent. *The Duke* cuts to the chase, through the rhetoric, and subtly redirects him to, "What ails you?"

His story is fairly unbelievable. He has been drinking with friends, (whose names he does not know) and he believes they have put some sort of poison---what type, he does not know---in his "Hennessy". He has drunk a lot of Hennessy and has never felt this bad. He denies any drug use, but reverses himself and admits to smoking some weed. In Austin, weed is akin to Cheerios, not drugs.

During "Poison Guy's" soliloquy, one of the Tac officers sticks his head in the side door and inquires as to any attitude problems. The boys assure him that everyone is playing nice. The Tac cop, who does not look like anyone you would ever want to fool with, says, "You better be nice or I'll be back." "Poison Guy" doesn't respond, but the message has been received, loud and clear.

Now, "Poison Guy" is insisting on going to the hospital, "So real Docs can check me out." He also admits that he really needs to get there so that he can convince his "old lady" that he has a good reason for being out this late. In the spirit of marital harmony, *The Duke* agrees and "Poison Guy" gets limoed over to West Suburban. When last seen, he was happily awaiting the results of his toxicology screen.

Run Number Sixteen/02:19 hrs: Number 15 rolls up on a *'woman with a diabetic problem'* call. An engine company and four firemen are inside where a non-responsive, elderly woman is in bed and doesn't look good on any level. DiGiovanni steps in and assumes control.

They are in a neat, well-kept, single family home where four intact generations of family live. The matriarch on the bed looks like she is about ten minutes from going to the funeral home as opposed to the ER. Also present is her elderly husband, her daughter, Mickey, (not her real name); Mickey's husband, Mickey's two daughters, and Mickey's grandchildren. Add six CFD guys and you have a jam-packed house. Unlike almost every other call 15 has responded to, these family members are somber and concerned. They are appropriate and normal. It is refreshing after a long day of bad attitudes and apathy.

Jay and Mike are working. Jay and Mickey discuss Grandma's health history, diabetes numbers, and all health-related issues that may be involved here. No one is excited, but everyone is anxious. No one wants to lose Grandma. Every possible effort will be made here. The firemen, who never look excited, are even displaying a little angst. This seemingly routine call has suddenly turned into a high stakes poker game.

Jay hardly breaks a sweat. Mickey and he have this figured out. Grandma is not fully conscious yet, but is starting to stir. Jay explains how Grandma can avoid being taken to the hospital, it boils down to one thing---Grandma has to get some carbs into her and it has to happen as soon as possible, preferably breakfast. Mickey does not have to be told twice. Pots and pans and bacon and eggs fly off the shelves. The men of the household all agree that breakfast is a great idea, so Mickey prepares a buffet.

Grandma has now been revived. She is conscious and coherent. She agrees to eat and admits that she is hungry. Mickey states that Grandma always eats well and diet is not an issue. Jay, Grandma, and Mickey decide that a trip to the hospital is not necessary or in her best interest. Jay gives explicit directions to Mickey who agrees to call if anything negative happens. She also promises that Grandma will be in her regular doctor's office first thing in the morning. Everyone agrees there is a need for a change in meds. CFD packs it all in and they depart happy.

From an outside observer, this appears to be miracle territory. Grandma was on death's door and she doesn't go to the hospital? DiGiovanni explains it was just a matter of getting some serious sugar into her quickly. "As soon as the sugar hit her, she came around. The family totally had their act together. Her care at home was first rate. I was not worried about follow up. Mickey knew as much about her mother's problems as does Grandma's doctor. She was in excellent hands. Normally, we would have taken her in, especially if the family was not really 'with it'. In this case it was not in her best medical interest to go in. It would not have been helpful."

Jay went on to say, "We have literally started cooking for victims while we've been on calls. The engine guys have actually started pulling out pots, pans and food and frying up breakfast. Sometimes that does more good than any medicine you can give them. There are times when we go out to buy groceries and come back after shift and make the kids some food. On the West Side, we get it done. There just isn't any manual for this stuff."

Buying groceries, cooking, learning and speaking medical Spanish? Boys and girls, *The Duke* is the whole package!

Run Number Seventeen/03:20hrs: *"15, victim with severe head pain."* It's off in the blowing, cold rain to a housing project with iron gates where you have to be let in. It takes a few minutes to find the right gate. All of them are locked. There's no access. Finally, a middle-aged guy comes running out in his boxers and lets the boys in. They enter the building and a stout

27-year-old woman, covered in tattoos, races down the stairs and says, "Y'all got to come up. I'm on a bracelet," then races back up the stairs. She does not look like she has severe head pain. Mike is not happy. "What she wants are some drugs and a way out without getting locked up for leaving home confinement." Mike returns to the ambo with the stretcher. Jay goes up and deals with the bracelet monitoring people. He has to tell them that he is taking their subject to the hospital.

This is about the only way that the woman can leave her apartment without getting locked up for violation of her parole or bond limitations. She knows it and 15 has seen this act before—a lot. Off to West Suburban they go. The woman isn't even trying to pretend that she's making this up. She is anticipating a trip to the ER and hopefully some good quality pharmaceutical drugs. She walks in under her own power. The boys spin around and are back in service before they hit the electronic doors. *The Duke* almost looks a little peeved. It's the closest he will get to being pissed off. *The Duke* never lets them know they are getting to him—not ever.

Run Number Eighteen/05:17 hrs: It's the longest break of the night. Jay puts his feet up in his private office and Mike pounds down some nicotine and coffee. He's gearing up for a twelve-hour shift at another side job after pulling 24 on this one. He's married, but does not have children yet. His wife works full-time, so he grabs the extra dough whenever he can. Jay says, "Man, Mike he never sleeps." Apparently not.

"15, man has fainted at YMCA." It's off to the YMCA building, which has been converted to a hotel for poor people who pay by the day. It's a quick trip and they only have to deal with about ten steps. They enter the lobby and a very slender well-dressed 59-year-old man is waiting for them next to a security guard who looks happy for any action.

Jay asks the man if he is ok. The man explains that he had passed out, but he came to before they got there. He complains of some sort of non-specific head pain. The boys help him into the ambo. The man explains, in broad, non-specific strokes, that he passed out last week and again this morning before they got there. Jay tries to get him to be more concise. Mike sniffs BS in the air, but says nothing. The man clearly wants to go to the hospital. He especially wants to go to West Suburban. Jay has to assure him three different times that they are, in fact, going to West Suburban. From the front, Mike says, "Cook County, right?"

The patient, who had been serenely lying on the stretcher with his hands folded on his chest and eyes closed, perks right up. "Nooo, West Suburban!" Jay says, "Don't worry, Sir, we're taking you to West." Mike silently protests by driving really slow.

Run Number Nineteen/06:11 hrs: It starts innocently enough. *"15, Asthma attack on West Lamon."* The boys are in hour twenty-three and after many years of working Austin they have the rhythm and pace down to a science. Internally, they are beat up. Outwardly there is no change. They look the same as they did on Run Number One. Jay looks a little worried. Asthma calls are sneaky deadly. You cannot let your guard down because it can turn to shit in the blink of an eye.

They quickly roll up on a woman in the street who is flagging them down. She is short and obese. The closer they get, the worse she looks. She comes right to the side door and Jay hauls her in. There is a real sense of urgency. Mike comes in right behind her. She is really laboring. She has the look of cold panic on her face, like someone who is drowning. Lake Michigan is about seven miles west, but that does not matter. She is drowning in her own fluids. Her lungs are in horrible shape. She is a lifelong asthmatic. This is not her first rodeo, but it might be shaping up to be her last.

Jay and Mike work without delay, in ultra-high gear. All of their skill sets rock in unison. The Klingon medical jargon pours out of them. The patient has that desperate "I am dying" look on her face. She gasps and fights for every breath. It is not pretty. Death seldom is, but this, this is something especially bad. You can smell it and taste it in the confined space of the ambo.

Jay has an oxygen mask on her before she sits down. He fires questions at her. She can only nod or weakly shake her head. There is not enough air in her to orally answer. Jay pumps inhaler into the oxygen mask and runs a stethoscope all over her chest and back. The right lung is not working. The left lung is barely hanging in there. More drugs, more questions. More nodding, shaking the head. She starts to come around a little. Mike has all the vitals down and the IV plugged in. They hit her with everything they have. This is as real as it gets.

Then it comes. Jay looks at her and softly says, "Honey, you do some heroin today?" She shakes her head no. Her eyes tear up. Everyone realizes all this might have, should have, been avoided. Jay says even more softly, "You do any yesterday?" She nods yes. Jay goes on, "One bag?" She shakes her head no. "Two bags?" She nods yes and leans back, starting to breathe easier. She has lost the drowning look. The boys slow it down. They have beaten the bastard death again.

It's a moment a civilian watching will never forget. For the boys, another day at the office. There is no celebration, no high fives. There should be something, but that will not happen in 15. They get the patient ready and transport her to West Suburban.

She gets handed off to the ER folks. There is no thank you or expression of gratitude. None are given and none are expected. For the ninetieth time in 24 hours, Jay starts the paperwork and Mike prepares the ambulance. They return to the firehouse where their relief crew is waiting.

The boys grab their personal bags and hand over Ambulance 15. Jay's relief paramedic asks, "Tough tour?" Jay responds, "Nothing special, pretty routine." Somewhere in the universe, Stan Zydlo is smiling. This is exactly what he envisioned. This paramedic juggernaut works exactly like he willed it to do.

Keeping Austin's People Alive

The unforgiving, seven and a half square mile area known as Austin consists of not much more than a mix of unemployment, apathetic schools, crime, drugs, institutional racism, and endemic cycles of poverty and disenfranchisement. Not many things work well, or as they should, in Austin.

Gang banging and drugs potentially offer a way out of the inane drudgery of daily life. In direct contrast to feelings of boredom, purposelessness, and insignificance, the street gangs offer redemption through the image of the urban warrior, recast as some sort of Robin Hood. The sad fact is nothing is further from the truth.

Lucky for the sick, crazy and deranged of the Austin community, Ambulance 15 is even better then the Duracell bunny and the city that never sleeps. It's always there when you need it. It doesn't bitch or complain or ask you to take out the garbage. It will not cheat on you or snitch you out to the man. It is, in short, the ultimate life preserver in a sea of lost hope and desperation.

Anywhere else in the western world, Jay DiGiovanni and Mike Kuryla might be getting department commendations for the past 24 hours of work and effort. Not in Austin, not on 15. *The Duke* neither requires or wants any official recognition. He only wants to keep his Austin people alive. That is why *The Duke* is as cool as the other side of the pillow and, day in and day out, perhaps Austin's most consistent valuable commodity. Long live *The Duke*.

CHAPTER ELEVEN

"Black Jack"

"There are more than 9,000 billing codes for
individual procedures and units of care."
– Clayton M. Christensen

The Innovator's Prescription: A Disruptive
Solution for Health Care

The economic impact of the paramedics and prehospital care, as Dr. Zydlo referred to it, is perhaps unmatched in its monetary effect on the U.S economy. Billions, if not trillions, of dollars in revenue have been generated simply because the paramedics save lives and then transport victims to the hospital alive. Ronald Reagan's chief budget guru, David Stockman, talked about 'trickle down' economics. This theory was that the more money people at the top of the money food chain made, the more that money trickled down to the rest of us. This never happened. It was a misguided theory that never performed as advertised. Think of the paramedic programs as 'trickle up' economics and you can bet the farm that this does trickle like a Tsunami drowns everything in its path. The trickle up starts immediately upon getting into an ambulance and arriving at the local emergency room. Whether you need five stitches for a cut, or you are having chest pains, look out. Hospital prices are arbitrary and punitive. There are no laws that regulate what can be charged. Arriving via ambulance is a hospital's wet dream. It is almost surprising that a marching band is not there to greet the next patient.

Given that most hospitals are not for profit entities and thus save hundreds of millions of dollars, or even more in tax breaks, don't think for one second those savings get passed on to the consumer. Quite the contrary. The goring and real bloodletting starts the second you are rolled into the emergency room. What you are charged is neither arbitrary nor connected to underlying costs, according to Professor Melnick, a leading economist. In short, there are no market constraints.[27]

Simply put, emergency room interventions are the mothers of all cash cows and, like all cash cows, this results in a nearly endless stream of cash flow depending upon how injures or sick you are. In 1993, more than thirty-seven million dollars in medical bills were generated in Chicago by the 2,500 people treated in emergency rooms for injuries inflicted by firearms.[28] In today's dollars, that figure is fifty-nine million dollars and change. That applies only to Chicago and only for gunshot victims.[29] This does not include cardiac events, vehicular accidents and the other situations that EMT/Paramedics get involved in every minute of every day. The hospitals, and subsequent medical personnel, who receive these patients have a stream of income that is damn near endless.

The hospitals counter with the argument that many of their patients are on some type of public assistance and therefore they are dependent upon the government to get paid and the government, of course, does not simply write a check for the full amount. The government actually sets the price point and pays that amount. The point is that the hospital will generally get paid by somebody, be it private insurance, government reimbursement via Medicaid, or a private individual, but generally a combination of the aforementioned.

Lest you begin to think that any hospital will do in an emergency, that is definitely not true. Fire department ambulances most always ship patients to the nearest trauma center. In the Chicago area, there are at least seven Level One hospitals. Where the patient ends up is often based on geography. How close is the nearest Level One facility? Do they have available staff to treat? Do they have enough beds available? On a busy summer weekend in Chicago, it is not uncommon for there to be fifty or sixty gunshot victims.

There is no way one hospital could handle that many patients, so they get spread out. In 2014, there were 2,587 gunshot victims in the city of Chicago. That averages out to around seven per day. The vast majority are shot during Friday through Sunday so that figure of seven a day does not tell the real story. Out of that 2,587 there were 435 dead. That does not reflect whether the dead died at the scene or died two weeks later, but for the sake of this discussion, that means that the paramedics saved 2,152 people.

We are not suggesting that the paramedics actually saved those people all by their lonesome, but they certainly had an impact on the vast majority of them that survived. Remember, this figure does not begin to cover the other lives saved by paramedic intervention performed in cardiac events, traffic accidents, choking, poisoning, allergic reactions, etc.

If you are shot, or have any need for an emergency service in the city of Chicago, this is what you can be expected to pay for a fire department ambulance.

Basic life support: $ 900.00
Advanced life support: $1,050.00

Advance life support II: $1,200.00

Oxygen: $ 25.00 (regardless of the amount)

Mileage*: $ 17.00 per mile

An additional fee of $100.00 shall be assessed for individuals who are not residents of the city of Chicago.

Any drugs used in the ambulance will be billed by the hospital because they supply the ambulance with all needed drugs. The consumer, not the fire department, picks up that bill, as well. If you get the feeling that this whole money issue is out of control, you are correct. However, the alternative is even less promising than the bill.

Looking back to 1971, when this whole paramedic thing was being created by Dr. Zydlo and the fire chiefs, the biggest concern in the medical community was that Zydlo's idea would start this country down the road to socialist medicine which is still pretty much heresy to the American medical community. In reality, the paramedic system started a financial bonanza that the bean counters in the medical community never envisioned. Don't fault the bean counters alone though because no one else anticipated or even guessed what financial riches were about to unfold.

Again, lest we think it is just doctors and hospitals getting wealthy, think again. Here is a smattering of the professionals involved in this medical lottery:

Nurses

Desk clerks

Admitting personnel

Janitors

Pharmaceutical companies

Manufacturers of equipment

Claims adjusters

Insurance industry

Medical labs

Bill collection agencies

Security and alarm companies

The list just keeps growing from the people who manufacture the light bulbs that are used in the ambulance to the companies that provide laundry services and sell bed sheets, blankets and Bandaids. How about the lawyers who represent the hospital, who sue the paramedics and fire departments, and the bill collection companies that are getting filthy rich specializing in medical collections only? The whole notion that this program would be free and wind up bankrupting emergency rooms, and consequently hospitals, is so ludicrous now that the reverse has occurred. Then there are the costs of these services that the hospitals never have to contribute a penny towards. None of this is inexpensive and this is just the tip of the financial commitment for the fire departments. They are:

Personnel and salaries

Ambulance

Workers comp and medical insurances for injuries

Medical equipment

Training

Support (squad-engine co.)

Computer and reports

What would happen on a financial level if the paramedics were not generating billions of dollars in fees and expenses? What would the economy look like then?

Zydlo had an idea about how all this would play out, but he never, ever, considered the financial boon that it would eventually become, mostly because that was not his area of interest and the fact that he was not involved in this concept for the sake of making money. Which leads us to the sad fact that the men and women who are actually out in the street risking life and limb are often paid less than that janitor in the hospital who mops up the mess.

Larger city fire departments generally pay very well with benefits and pension packages, but even the good pay at those departments does not begin to cover the thousands of men and women who do this on a volunteer level. Medium to small jurisdictions often pay substantially less and, finally, some rural areas are all volunteer and those people are paid zero for their services.

The trend today is that small and medium sized towns, cities, and rural fire districts are merging, eliminating jobs and overhead. Once again, the paramedics and EMTs are hammered professionally and personally. It is nothing short of criminal that this is happening on a large, nationwide scale. Politicians are gutting their pensions and perks, while sliding the savings over to their own pensions, benefits, and salary. Yet, some cities are *eliminating their fire departments* and hiring private contractors. In some Chicago suburbs, the paramedics are working 48 hour shifts in an effort to save money. What about the paramedics? What kind of long-term effect is this having on them? Their families? Their physical well-being? Last, but not least, is patient care. No one is answering those questions.

This national trend is beyond disgraceful. The one service provided to the public, to the poor, the wealthy, the mentally deficient, homeless, drunk, and stupid on an equal basis is getting screwed in a major way. The paramedic industry is under attack and, typical of people who perform these services, they are not prepared to respond appropriately to protect themselves and their families. Not because they are incapable of doing so, but that is not what they do, or who they are. That is not in their collective nature and their mindset is always to respond, serve, and protect.

Very few of these people are in this business for the economic rewards. Most, if capable, would work for free if that is what it took, but when you have a family you are not allowed that luxury. The tragedy here is the pending disaster from fooling around with, and systematically gutting, one of the rare programs that actually functions like it is supposed to is happening now and getting worse.

As with all things political, you have politicians making decisions that affect a large section of the population. Therein lies the problem. The political masters who are seldom interested in anything beyond enriching themselves, getting re-elected, and raising money, are screwing around with a system that is about as nearly perfect as anything can be. Toss in the uber-wealthy hospitals and their money mercenaries who run those institutions and you have the perfect storm brewing. If the fire departments and paramedics don't wake up and start getting proactive in these matters, it could be the start of the death march of their profession as they know it.

You will likely not hear any talk of these matters from anyone who manages or has a financial stake in a hospital. Nevertheless, an excellent starting point is what happens when you get carted off to the nearest hospital after an emergency or serious incident. In 2014, in Florida, the state average ER cost was $4,546. North Florida Regional Medical Center in Gainesville had the highest average charge in Florida at a whopping $11,413 per ER visit in 2014. Only three hospitals had an average charge of $1,000 or less. Complexity and seriousness of the visit vary from hospital to hospital.[30]

The National Institute of Health funded a study in 2013 and the results were staggering. Nationwide, the average ER visit will cost you or your insurance company on average $1,233.00 for one visit. That figure is higher than forty percent of the average monthly rent bills in the U.S, which is $871.00. There are huge variations in price. The researchers found bills for sprained ankles that had a low of four dollars and a high of $24,110. Patients with no medical coverage often pay more money than those who have it.[31]

At one time, hospital ER bills were not out of control. People, in general, were happy with services provided there. Not anymore. People are horrified at the shenanigans. Copied below are some randomly selected complaints:

"This hospital did excessive testing when all I needed was six stitches. I repeatedly told her that I just needed my lip sewn up. The result was a $40,000 bill I can't pay. That seems quite a lot for six stitches. As a result, I could not refinance my home so that I might lower the payment. My family and I are struggling money-wise like everyone else."

"I came in with blisters on my hand, mouth and feet. All they did was a swab of my mouth and blood work. I was not given any medicine (just a prescription for mouthwash) and told I had hand-foot-and-mouth disease. I am very out done at the charges. I was charged for 2-3 hours. And on my bill they never described what I was charge $15,020.00 for. Nothing stating they charged me $3,000 for blood work just a flat bill owing $15,020.00. That's a very ridiculous price for what I was seen for."

"The hospital billed me for $12,745.44. I owe $9,559.08 for a kidney stone. I think that is a bit much."

"Tripped and fell in my driveway and broke left cheekbone and other bones on left side. Driven by my sister to emergency room. We were told they don't treat trauma cases and I was sent to another hospital 50 miles away

by ambulance, but not before they sent me to radiology for x-ray and CT scans. I was there about two hours. My bill for being uninsured was over 15K. Almost 10K of which was radiology. I have another approximately 4K in separate charges for ER doctor; $1,500, $880 to read x-rays, $740 for two-hour ambulance ride. There are a couple others amounting to about another $1,000. I was in shock but told them I was uninsured and do not remember signing any papers in the condition I was in."[32]

This is just a tiny sample of how the American public is being fleeced. The entire system is upside down and people are drowning under the weight of debt. A Harvard study from 2007 indicates that at least 60% of all bankruptcies are medical bill related. In 2007, the Commonwealth Fund discovered that seventy-two million Americans are struggling with medical bills.[33]

In 2014, there were 936,795 bankruptcies filed nationally. That translates into almost 500,000 of them being medical bill related.[34] That is a whole lot of federal courtroom time being tied up. It is also very profitable for the lawyers and personnel required to be involved in the case by statute. No one working for free.

So where does this mega type lottery money wind up? What is the final destination of these gargantuan profits? Simply put, the end game is expansion. Expansion of the emergency room. Expansion of the cardiac center, laboratories, X-Ray, MRI, and CAT scan departments. Expansion of the hospital in general. Bigger is better and even bigger than bigger is better yet.

None of this happens in a vacuum, by chance or accident. It is the cumulative effort of the genius and experience of some very driven and often brilliant people.

On a practical level, these issues are often decided on a cost-benefit analysis, (CBA).[35] Why do the CBA at all since there are so many imponderables? The CBA is often the driving force in any governmental decision. The other is politics and in this specific case, thank God for small miracles, because if these decisions were based on the CBA, Chicago Ambulance #15 would not exist in today's bottom line driven world of bean counters.

We may not like hearing about the CBA, but when making serious financial decisions, the City of Chicago will never *not* consider the CBA.

It would be magnificent if there was an Ambulance #15 on every corner. There is no telling how many more lives would be saved. A great theory, but at what expense are we willing to do this? You want the sacred cow budget items? Who is going to vote to reduce teacher salaries? How about snow removal? Are you going to remove snow and salt the streets on even numbered days? What about the garbage? Who has the political balls to charge extra for garbage removal? Oh, wait—the City has done just that.

Be that as it may, the evil CBA is a fact of life. There are always political and real ramifications when budget dough is spread around. No one agency gets everything it wants. Well, maybe the IRS and Homeland Security, but everyone else is forced to live in the real world---especially the fire department and its EMS budget.

This begs the valid question of what is a human life worth? To say the least, that date is fluid. Who would be stupid enough to *put* a number on that equation? You will be shocked, but "Yes" your very own government has hammered away with your tax dollars to answer that very question.

The vast majority of developed nations put the figure at $50,000 per year of quality-adjusted life. That figure was generated by the cold, black, collective hearts of the insurance industry in a paid study subsidized by them. The Department of Transportation pegs it at six million. The Food and Drug Administration, in a 2010 study, says $7.9 million. The

Environmental Protection Agency states $9.1 million. That was in 2008. *TIME* magazine says $129,000.

Given that characterization of the challenge, one might expect to hear that approximately 30,000 people die in car accidents in the United States each year. Close to zero would die if the government reduced the speed limit to 13 miles per hour. But do you want that to happen? Probably not.

In the medical community, qualitative expressions dominate medical decision-making terminology. You hear and read terms like "meaningful life," "prevailing interest," and "persistent vegetative state." Hospitals speak to the bottom line mentality when they talk about the necessity for "rationing." Rationing occurs when health care providers intentionally choose not to provide care to everyone who needs it. This is almost never spoken about out loud.

Where does the slippery slope end or stop? Do we have mandatory abortions for children with Down Syndrome? Do we overdose terminal cancer patients over the age of 75? How about 65 or 55? Do we move on to victims of brain injuries, MS, Cerebral Palsy? Prisoners with life sentences, or sex offenders?

It is all very arbitrary. The voluminous Talmud (Jewish Law) weighs in on the subject with the following: "There are two crucial principles. Firstly, that every individual human life has absolute, not relative, value. One times absolute is just as absolute as 10,000 times absolute. Seventy years of absolute value is just as absolute as one year or one hour of absolute value.[36]

This, of course, leads to the second economic tier that trickles uphill against the tide. The corporate owners of these health centers make no small plans. As smart as Zydlo was, he never saw this one coming. He certainly understood the immediate monetary rewards. "Get them there alive and everyone who is involved will make more money." He never dreamed of the second phase. The types of people and professions that get rich on these hospital expansions are as long as the one for medical-related personnel. To name a few:

Architectural firms

Construction companies and their subcontractors

Law firms

Governmental bodies like the EPA, local zoning and permit boards

Steel and building materials companies

Labor unions

Bank and bond companies

Insurance companies

Public relations and crisis management firms

For example, the University of Chicago Hospital recently proposed a major expansion in trauma service and their emergency room to the tune of 269 million dollars.[37] Neither the University of Chicago, nor any other major health care provider, lays out that kind of dough because they expect to lose money.

They do it for one reason and that is to *make money* and a lot of it. The level of sophistication that goes into making these financial decisions is not undertaken lightly. Prior to one shovel entering the dirt, one brick being laid, millions are spent just getting to the point of making a financial decision of that nature.

Very serious people, who do not generally make mistakes, make these decisions. If they do err, they don't last long. Yet at the end of the day, this venture is going to rise or fall directly on the backs of those paramedics in the street who are saving lives and getting the cash cow (patient) to the temple of dough and health care in good enough shape so that some of the 269 million dollars can be recovered. The most critical cog in this juggernaut is, of course, Zydlo's band of brothers and sisters who are most certainly the most abused and underappreciated in the whole process.

If any thought is given to the role of the paramedics in this grand scheme of greed and money grabbing, it is one of "How do we make sure that we are getting our fair share of patients from the fire department?"

Very little, if any, consideration is given to the treatment of the men and women who make the dream become a reality. "Not our problem." "They don't work for us." All true, but if the paramedics are going to stem the flow of their own bleeding and save themselves from the money changers at the temple, they better figure out how they can protect the brotherhood, the professions, and, of course, the people they serve.

Perhaps if the paramedics and ambulances shut down for one week, the communities they serve would take a little bit better care of them, but that will never happen because that is not who these people are. These are very real problems happening right now in every city. Ignoring these issues and hoping the masters will be benevolent and fair didn't work for the Irish, the slaves, or the labor unions. The end game is predictable and the only people who can save this magnificent system of prehospital care are the ones trolling in the trenches. We better all hope and pray they do.

CHAPTER TWELVE

"Do Overs"

"Remember…even if everything is wrong in your life today, as long as you are alive, you will always get another chance to start over tomorrow. A new beginning…a new dream…a new hope"
– Ash Sweeney

We give very little thought to what it means to have the opportunity at another shot at saving our marriage, to right a wrong we committed, or just simply to be a better person tomorrow, to live a more meaningful life. We get caught up in paying bills, hustling the kids from one event to another, getting to work, earning a living, finding the time to do a thousand little things that need doing every day and every hour of our lives. There is never enough time.

In the United States, 4,237 people will die of a heart attack today. If you're one of those four thousand plus people who drop dead from a heart attack tomorrow morning while you're working out on the treadmill, none of this will matter. However, if the health club gets an ambulance to you quick enough and the paramedics are competent enough to shock you back to life and get you to a trauma center where angioplasty can clean out those martini and steak-filled arteries, you will have a shot, a *do-over*. If thirty-six hours later you are home eating poached salmon and steamed broccoli while watching bad TV, maybe you should say a little prayer of thanks to Stan Zydlo and those "Zydlo-trained" paramedics who just bought another twenty years for you to repair your dysfunctional life.

So, looking backwards with a critical, historical eye, only one conclusion comes to mind: Dr. Zydlo and his "jack booted socialist paramedics" are responsible for more second chances than a Hindu Swami handing out reincarnation chits to twenty million other Hindus.

If you consider how many saved lives and the residual effects for friends and loved ones of those who would almost certainly be dead if not for Zydlo and the paramedics, you begin to get the idea of just how big this 'paramedic thing' has become. There is simply no other area of medicine that has impacted the world population more. Every person you know has a story of this nature. There is nowhere one can go and not find someone who hasn't had their life saved, or had the life of a loved one or friend saved by these incredibly gifted, modern day heroes. This is how big the paramedic program has become. There will never be anything imaginable that will replace or duplicate its success. That is how impactful this has become and that is why Dr. Stanley M. Zydlo, Jr. should be remembered as one of American's greatest heroes.

The following stories are examples of lives saved when all odds were against the injured person. Remember, also, the stories in the Paramedics chapter of Paramedics Kemper and Collier saving lives in Palatine, Illinois, and of Paramedic Kemper saving the lives of child passengers on a school bus hit by a train.

Miracle Man

You get up, brush your teeth, wolf down a bagel, throw some water on your face, and out the door you go to catch the bus for school. You've done it five hundred times. Easy-peasy baby, time to chat up that hot chick from English class. "Maybe she'll go to homecoming with me." Such are the world weary problems of a fifteen-year-old high school sophomore.

Your older sister offers you a ride on the way to her EMT class. She is a volunteer firefighter and sweet to ask, but she can't compete with the English class girl. "No thanks, Sis. I'll rough it on the bus." Off you go and that little half-second of thought process that had you pass on Sis's ride will change your life forever.

Man, you're on that bus and one second you're making some not so subtle goo-goo eyes with the English class girl and the next second the whole fucking world explodes like the worst IED bomb to go off in Iraq in the past ten years. Except this isn't Iraq and you're not a soldier in a combat zone. Nope, this is Cary Grove, Illinois and you are sitting on a school bus that just got t-boned by a commuter train going seventy-plus miles per hour.

As we have seen throughout history, and certainly in this story, life does and can turn in a millisecond. You're an adult. You lick your wounds and keep on marching because there is no other option. You presumably, (if you're not a total bust out) have a family, a career, children, and other adult-like responsibilities that are bigger than whatever your current little I-tune/Facebook, track is playing in that dysfunctional mess you call a mind. As an adult you have presumably mastered enough basic skills to survive a tragedy of this nature. But a fifteen-year-old hormonal, teen-aged boy? That is entirely a different cat and events of this nature could destroy him emotionally, and in effect, anyone else who at a later date is silly enough to think that they can "fix" his problems.

This was the defining moment for young Jason Kedrok. When the collision occurred, Jason was seated about a half foot away from being obliterated into a bloody, fine pink mist. For most young men, this event had enough firepower to wreak havoc on the strongest of souls. For Jason, this was just another disaster that followed one that had happened two weeks to the day when his father dropped dead. Jason, my friends, was not having a good month.

Jason's physical injuries were not serious, but for eight of his unlucky classmates and their families, this was the ultimate disaster where the loss of those young, bright-eyed eight lives destroyed a community and wreaked unimaginable pain and havoc on hundreds of friends and family. These are the types of events that define us and set in motion our life's path.

You can either sink (who would blame you?), tread water (just go through the motions and take up space), or you can gut check through it and have a meaningful life. Jason Kedrok, like Paramedic Ed Kemper, who jumped on the wrecked bus and saved many lives, took the latter path.

Fireman/Paramedic Captain Jason Kedrok is now thirty-six years old and an eight-year veteran of the Arlington Heights Fire Department, as well as a captain in the Fox River Grove, Illinois Volunteer Fire Department. He has stacked up a pretty nice resume in the brotherhood saving lives and showing up when it counts. Kedrok, who has experienced about as much grief as any human should be asked to live through, has done a mite more than just show up. More on that later.

Kedrok, who is the father of four, all under the age of six, is happily married and still living in the community in which he grew up. It would seem that maybe being a full-time fireman/paramedic and captain of *two* fire departments would keep Jason busy enough, but like many of our heroes chronicled here, he does nothing small. In addition to the starting five at home who presumably require attention on occasion, Jason and his wife also own a company that repairs fire equipment. Did I mention that he is also a certified and trained diesel mechanic who is the full-time mechanic for the Round Lake Beach Fire Protection District in northern

Illinois? Last, but not least, he also teaches fire science at a local community college. Jason apparently does not require sleep or nourishment.

In the history of second chances, it would appear that Jason Kedrok has certainly made the most of his second chance. You could even argue that he has taken advantage of his second chance like few others. But, even then when we dig deep and we think that Jason has done as well as anyone would have guessed, there is still more. Because when Fireman/Paramedic Ed Kemper jumped on that dissected, destroyed bus on that fateful day, the first kid, and in his mind, the most memorable one he came in contact with, was Jason Kedrok.

Kemper's memory of the event always returns to Jason because, as he says, Jason "was the first kid I saw and I had him round up the walking wounded and get them all off the bus and isolated so we could get them out faster." Kemper says that after that he got the more critically injured off the bus and the dead removed, the first thing recalled seeing was fifteen-year-old Jason standing exactly where he told him to go. He was watching and helping his classmates. Kemper (who is a Medal of Honor winner, and all around bad ass medic) was almost struck dumb by the maturity and selflessness displayed by Kedrok and, as a result, became a lifelong mentor and friend to him.

Arguably one of the bravest human beings walking amongst the rest of mere humans, Kemper has never forgotten that moment. Ironically, Jason suffered a pretty nasty concussion and a bad case of shock that day and remembers very little. This would be a nice ending for this story, but there is just a bit more.

As with many of the people in these pages, there always seems to be addendum to their own miraculous story. In Jason Kedrok's case, there are many noteworthy ones, but for him, two stand out. When Jason was asked to comment on any difficult or noteworthy, lifesaving acts he has been involved in personally, he, just like the rest of the heroic individuals in this book, minimized his actions.

Most of us understand the mechanics of these brave acts. We all realize that there are generally any number of people involved in these life-saving activities and our intent is not to diminish their role(s), but there is almost always one individual on a team who does the exact right thing at the critical second.

In Jason's case, there was the young, twenty-something-year-old woman who was shot in the head in a drug deal gone bad. When they rolled up, none of the emergency personnel on the scene thought she was alive. You can imagine the chaos, the blood, the gore, and smells that civilians will never understand or experience. In this case, though, Jason was either too young, or too inexperienced to pack it in and call the coroner. He went to work on her and the gunshot victim was not only pulled through, she survived with very little noticeable damage.

Jason's last, but hardly his most heroic, or even a top ten finalist, was in reality a simple, fairly pedestrian paramedic act that he will always carry with him no matter how ugly or hectic it gets out there. It was a cold, winter night in one of those barren, frosty cornfields that dot the Midwestern landscape. A young couple on the side of the road needed help and they needed it right now.

Remember Dr. Zydlo's mantra: "People need help when they need it." On that cold, blustery winter night, Jason Kedrok delivered his first baby as a paramedic and to those of you reading this, that might sound pretty boring and routine. Certainly just about every paramedic around has successfully pulled it together and delivered at least one child on the job. But for Jason, the father of four young kids, this was HUGE! If you are feeling let down with Jason's accomplishment, ask yourself one question---"What would have happened if Jason Kedrok had not been there?"

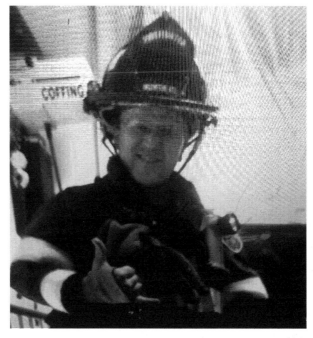

Arlington Heights IL Paramedic/Firefighter Jason Kedrok, Circa 2015.
Courtesy Jason Kedrok

Third and long. Real long…

So it is appropriate that we close this real life drama, and the bread and butter of lifesaving actions which is simply, any cardiac-related event. Paramedics respond to every conceivable accident and medical emergency call that you can think of. They respond to every call and they almost always do what they are supposed to do. But if there is one medical emergency that could ever be considered "routine" it is any occurrence involving a heart attack type event.

Early on in the late '60s and early '70s, when forward thinking medical professionals were kicking this whole EMT/Paramedic idea around, it was driven by medical emergencies involving cardiac events. This was mostly due to a number of factors, but the overriding consensus was heart attacks were, and will always be, the number one cause of death, if not treated without delay.

If a well-trained and equipped ambulance shows up while you are in the middle of the old chest gripper and they get there before you have quit breathing for six minutes or more and the paramedics are on their "A" game, you have a pretty decent chance of living to fight another day, to have a second chance at life.

An extraordinary amount of time, effort, and money, is spent in training EMS personnel and the continuing education of EMS personnel to competently and successfully treat individuals who are experiencing a cardiac event. These events drove the early march towards the complete and totally competent EMS programs and it remains relevant today. Many of the men and women in this book have been the beneficiaries of a well-trained colleague who was also a paramedic.

On two separate occasions, Zydlo-trained paramedics saved Dr. Zydlo when he had heart attacks at home. Now retired, Rolling Meadows Chief and Paramedic Ted Loesch saved former Rolling Meadows Fire Chief Tom Fogarty when he went down with a heart attack in his home one morning. Finally, Schaumburg EMS Coordinator and former paramedic, Steve Johnson's life was saved when he suffered a massive heart attack while working out in the firehouse gym many years ago.

Tragedy and medical events happen every second of every day and one never knows when the fickle finger of fate will point in your direction. So we end this with the almost tragic ending of Michael Bertschinger. Michael needed serious help on June 2, 2013 when he was driven up to the Schiller Park, Illinois firehouse located a stone's throw from Chicago's O'Hare airport.

Born and raised in the Omaha, Nebraska area, Mike was pretty much living the dream. Good looking, smart, gifted three sport athlete, college educated, great job, hot girlfriend…well, you get the idea. The world was his oyster. He had worked hard and diligently to get where he was. Some people would call Mike "lucky".

The fact is, he made his own luck and had done all he could to be successful in life. The youngest of four siblings raised in a close knit, middle class, working family, he seldom drank, and had never smoked. At six foot two, and a well-defined 190 pounds, he watched his diet and worked out religiously. At the time of his incident, he was in a stable relationship living together with his girlfriend in Chicago's south loop neighborhood. He was a successful marketing executive with a national company and his life could not have been going much better than it was when he got up that bright Sunday morning in June.

It was a little cool for June with temperatures in the mid-50s and clear. He felt like a million bucks. He was amped up because he was playing in a competitive men's adult flag football league single elimination, championship tournament, in Schiller Park, Illinois. This was not a beer league where overweight, out of shape, former high school football players kick it around and have a good time. This was a serious league in which serious, really athletic studs played.

They were all gifted athletes and good enough to win a U.S.A. championship. Mike had played football through college, a wide receiver with great speed. For a white guy, he could flat out fly. He loved everything about football—the competition, the camaraderie, the physical aspects and the smell of fresh cut grass. It was, and always had been, his game, his greatest stress reliever.

He had always been cautious about his health. Never had any health-related issues. Not a one, until that fine June morning. It started simply enough. He had just run a simple route, caught the ball, and scored. He was walking out of the end zone when he felt a slight chest pain. Nothing serious, more of a twinge than a pain. That game ended. As he walked over to the field to start the next game, Bam! It started with a burning sensation in his chest and got progressively worse by the second.

Michael Bertschinger. Who would have thought this guy would have a massive, almost deadly, heart attack?

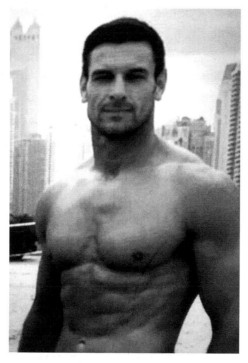

Mike Bertschinger, Date unknown, Courtesy of Mike Bertschinger

He thought it was an "air thing." It was a little cool, almost frosty for June. They were right next to one of the world's busiest airports and not the greatest air quality around. He stopped and bent over, taking deep breaths trying to get more air and oxygen down. Now people were starting to look at him, asking if he was okay. He waved them off. "yeah, I'm good guys."

Wishful thinking. He was anything but "good," he just didn't know how bad it would get in about ten minutes. There was one fan present that day, the father of one of Mike's teammates. That was it. Sixty, seventy grown men running around playing football and there was exactly one fan present, a dad. Not a doctor or a medic dad, just your run of the mill, middle-aged, crusty Chicago dad with nothing better to do on a cool June morning. Crusty Dad walked over to Mike, took one look at him and says, "Hey, you ain't looking too good. Let's go get you checked out."

Mike, in a state of denial at this point and, unbeknownst to him, starting to lose oxygen along with common sense, said, "I'll be okay in a minute."

Bullshit. Now the pain was really kicking in and Mike knew something was desperately wrong. He's hoping against hope, but his oxygen-deprived brain is unable to recognize that he's in serious trouble. He starts to sweat profusely and turns pale. Crusty Dad has seen enough. He grabs Mike by the arm, walks him over to his car, and puts him in the front seat. No one else is paying much attention, but Crusty Dad is, and Michael is feeling more dog shit by the second. Now, there is no doubt he is in deep waters and sucking air. The thought, "heart attack" has not entered the fog of his mind yet, but it would soon enough.

Crusty Dad is worried. This really good looking, in shape kid, sure as shit looks like he's having a heart attack. How in the hell is that possible? He looks frigging great except for the fact he looks like he's about to drop dead. The pain, the sweats, no air and Michael figures he's dying and he has no idea why. He has never experienced anything close to this. He can hardly talk. He's bent over in the front seat of Crusty Dad's car. His sense is that Crusty Dad is driving faster and faster. He can feel movement, but his vision starts to go. Suddenly, they are in a parking lot, a firehouse parking lot, right in front of the big doors.

He was the good son. He was low maintenance. He was an excellent athlete who got a football scholarship to college. His Dad was a guy, who when he was younger, went on vacation with him. He was never home and, let's face it, his mother was the rock. She did it all and he and his brothers and sister knew it. The old man, he was great when he was home, but that was like every three months or so. He worked like a dog and he had a job like no other dad that he was aware of.

The old man was a star. Every social event, school event, football game, he attended, he was always the center of attention. He was a flame that all the moths flew to. The son would watch all this. He would observe and say little. The father was a keen observer of human behavior. He knew this kid out of all his children was a pisser. He didn't say much, but he missed nothing. He was a straight A student and could probably do anything he wanted to do. He wasn't saying, but the old man definitely did not want the kid in the family business.

Inside the firehouse, there is another thirty-one-year-old male. He played linebacker at a prestigious Catholic Prep high school outside of Chicago. One of his teammates was the son of Hall of Fame Chicago Bears running back Walter Payton. The fireman loved football. He played in college on a scholarship until his knee got destroyed in practice. Goodbye, Division One, hello fire department.

In reality, he didn't want to be anywhere else. He loved his job. He loved saving lives. He loved the little kids he ran into. He loved the firehouse life, the closeness of his colleagues. Football was great. It taught him much. It helped develop his leadership skills. He just loved knocking the shit out of a quarterback. But he really loved saving lives. That was a rush. Bringing someone back from the brink---that was real, grownup fun. That was meaningful and it gave him instant gratification. From the depths of his worldview, that was how he saw it.

He also grew up in a large family. He was exceptionally bright. He thought about attending medical school at certain points. He had the grades and the chops, but his parents were not encouraging. They did not want him working that hard. They wanted him to have a life that didn't entail killing yourself every day.

He became a paramedic. Schiller Park eventually hired him after he had held a number of similar positions. They love him and he loves the job. It's a great match and he is stable, happy and accomplished. At Schiller Park, every fireman is a certified paramedic. Everyone's an expert, even if they have not worked an ambulance for ten years.

His shift starts at 0900hrs, but he is always there by eight. Starts his paperwork, talks to the guys on the shift he's relieving, and then gets ready for roll call. It's a comfortable, predictable way to start the day. Kind of lets one ease into the shit storm that will happen at any moment. It's not *if*, but *when* it kicks off. You work a busy house. There is never a dull moment. By virtue of this profession, every call is an emergency. Every call your body is reacting.

It is high stressful and make you get old far before your time. There are a lot of burnouts, divorces, alcohol and drug problems. The list is never ending and it's almost all bad. He would not, no, could not, do anything else. This was his life and he would not change one thing. He thinks, "Man, I was born to do this shit." He was. At this particular moment in life, in this little speck on a really big map, the young paramedic was exactly where he should be.

In about two minutes there will be a huge collision. Two men in the prime of their lives are going to run into each other. Both come from fairly large families. Both were excellent students and athletes. Both played college football. Both are good looking, but neither of them can predict what will happen. It will be one of those things that are life-changing. It is the stuff of the Cosmos, Karma, or is it God intervening in earthly events, or just a mere coincidence? Who can really say, but both of these young men will be vastly different people within an hour after meeting

Things are not improving in Crusty Dad's car. Michael is certain he is near death. All he can think about is how this will screw up his whole family. He blames himself for something that is entirely not of his making. Nevertheless, in the fog of his brain he is thinking how badly his family will take this. It is ripping him up and there is not a damn thing he can do about it. He is sad beyond words. He is not thinking about his life, his losses, just devastated over how his parents and siblings will react. He does not want them to suffer. He is just stricken by the whole idea. He is not considering his own demise.

Crusty Dad had his foot buried in the carburetor. All of those "Dad senses" are screaming in his head. He knew the minute he laid eyes on this young man something was seriously fucked up. His instincts, his subconscious, all recognized it before he did. He did not want to believe that this seemingly healthy looking young stud was about to drop dead. He didn't want to deal with it, but the "Dad senses" were doing what great dads do every day and that was using his instinct and gut feelings to save future younger dads from themselves.

He was flat out flying and in the urban desert of a small industrial suburb of Chicago, there was the oasis. Right in front of him, on his right--the well of life, the answer to his prayers. A firehouse! A big, old shitty looking building of brick and mortar. Crusty Dad knew one things for certain. This was better than the hospital. This was the game changer that this young dude next to him needed.

Crusty Dad wheeled into that parking lot at about sixty miles per hour and was out of the car before it stopped. He was no athlete, but he moved like Audie Murphy through the Germans. He thought as he dashed into the building, "Not today death, you Mother F'er. You are not winning today."

Inside, our young paramedic was just finishing some paperwork when he heard the commotion in the parking lot. "Uh, oh," he thinks. "I know that sound. That is the sound of shit hitting the fan and it's not a birthday cake delivery or a singing stripper for someone's birthday". (Not that strippers have ever been in a firehouse in this country, but when you're young, you can hope.) No, this was the sound of someone in big trouble. They only drove up like that when someone was in deep shit.

Immediately, the training kicked into high gear. The adrenaline rush starts to surge and shits and giggles time screamed to a stop. It was all business now and every paramedic/firefighter in the house was off their ass and charging towards the shit storm that is now Michael Bertschinger's immediate reality. There was no hesitation, no wasted effort. It was a grand, beautiful symphony of movement and greatness honed by thousands of similar incidents and training. Crusty Dad and Mike have no clue, but they just may have hit the winning lottery ticket.

Mike can still talk and move a little. Shit moves at warp speed now. Stretchers fly out of the back of the parked ambulance. Guys in blue work clothes grab him and put him on the board. A good looking female paramedic fires questions at him and he feels a little guilty for thinking the good looking thought, but he can't help himself. Talent is talent no matter how close you are to death.

The young fireman prays it's not a young kid in trouble. He has a child at home and every time he deals with a baby or toddler, he thinks of his kid. Those are the tough ones. The next worst are the young, healthy dudes and dudettes. Young, healthy people are not supposed to die. You don't want to lose a young cat. Sure enough, it's his second worst case scenario. It's a young guy and he looks like hell. Pale, struggling to breathe, definitely look bad and getting worse by the second.

Mike had been a fire cadet and a volunteer fireman in Nebraska. He wasn't a stranger to this dance. He still had some wits about him and understood on a cerebral level what was happening. For the first time, it dawned on him that he might be having a heart attack. A FRIGGING HEART ATTACK! Are you shitting me? Mr. health freak, work out maniac, don't smoke, don't drink, *that* dude was having a heart attack? *Me?*

It was rolling now. That big, old, fat, nasty blood clot was moving and heading straight for the old bull's eye. Right at the old ticker. There was no delay. It had a mind of its own and was moving like a heat seeking missile. It was doing its job. Everything around it was reacting. The lungs labored and were in overdrive trying to work, failing miserably. Kidney and liver function were sluggish. The heart was in the fight of its relatively young life, the brain turning to sludge. It was almost there.

The young paramedic, along with a couple of his colleagues, had Mike in the ambo now. They worked it. Everyone had a job. Not much talk, hanging IVs, popping some aspirin into Mike's mouth, hooking up a quarter million dollars of equipment to the patient. The rest of the shift was standing there watching, judging, evaluating. They rocked this shit and they knew it.

The first monitor hooked up responded immediately. There that bitch was. Bam! A huge S/T elevation. That means one thing---myocardial infarction, for you civilians, a heart attack. The big one. The old gripper. Mike's body, his old pal, was betraying him

The young fireman had this shit down cold. If he excelled at one thing, this was it. Heart attacks were his forte. He knew all the stats and all the protocols…by heart. He didn't need a book. He knew them like he knew the curve of his wife's rear end. What he knew for certain is that he had a young, healthy, white male lying in front of him and he was technically dead at the moment. The equipment does not lie. This guy was screwed. He had pulled up to the firehouse with about a five percent chance of survival. They hovered around zero chance at the moment.

In quick order, the paramedics hooked up twelve electronic leads to Mike. Every one of them is elevated. That means one thing---widow maker time. This is it. The heart is in V-Fib and shutting down. Mike has quit breathing. He has no pulse. The angel of death is lounging on top of his chest and it is game over for Michael Bertschinger. This was it. A life well-lived snuffed out. It had fought the fight and lost.

The left anterior descending artery was now one hundred percent blocked. This was it, no blood to the heart. The old pumper was not pumping anything. If this happens anywhere but an operating room in a trauma center, say goodbye, adios, sayonara baby. All that's left to do is to pick out the suit for the funeral.

Not today. Not in the back of the young paramedic's ambulance! Today, the linebacker was playing offense. No way he given this dude up. He's blasting the quarterback, grabbing the ball and taking it in for a TD with no time on the clock. The young paramedic snatched the paddles and slammed them into Mikes chest and yells, "Clear!" Bam. The electric shock slams into Mike with the force of Mike Tyson, in his prime, pounding a heavy bag.

Everyone watched the monitors. One of the paramedics had bagged Mike to force air down his mouth into his lungs. Mike's eyes fluttered open and he actually looked semi-coherent. The paramedic who had bagged him, leaned over and said in his best Chuck Yeager pilot voice, "We had a problem with your heart, but we fixed it."

Did that dude just say, "We fixed your HEART?" My heart! The dude sounded like he was talking about a flat tire. Mike was shocked. He was in zero pain. The gravity of the situation started to dawn on him as they pulled into the hospital and were greeted by a huge welcoming committee of doctors, nurses and other staff in the sally port.

They were expecting a dead man. The back doors of the ambo open and it's a flurry of activity. They wheeled Mike into the emergency room where the real expensive shit started. Tests, tests and more tests. Cat scans, blood draws, the full force of a modern, urban hospital teems with activity. It's doing exactly what Stan Zydlo designed it to do.

Michael Bertschinger will be okay. They got him into a CAT lab and inserted a huge tube into the femoral artery of his groin. They blasted the blood clot out, put in some stents and in less than seventy-two hours, Mike was sitting on his couch in the south loop of Chicago, watching ESPN and feeling none too worse for the wear and tear.

In a quiet moment after the adrenaline-filled rush of saving another human being's life, the young fireman was coming off that super charged feeling you get on the hot runs. He started to calm down. His pulse slowed and he breathed easier. His blood pressure was almost normal again. This was not his first save, but he knew it would always be a memorable one because of the age of the victim, the obvious signs of good health, the massive adrenaline dump experienced when a victim shows up at your doorstep.

There was no time to mentally prepare. No ride to an accident scene. No dialog with 911, the ER, or with his partner. Dude walked up to the firehouse and dropped like a ton of bricks right at your feet. Man, it happens in the blink of an eye. One minute you're kicking back BS'ing with the boys, working a crossword puzzle, watching the news, whatever. Two seconds later, you are slaying the death dragon.

You rip the guy's shirt off, trying to find a pulse. ("fuck me, no pulse/ zero blood pressure/zero signs of life, fuck, fuck, fuck this dude is frigging dead") You look cool. You got a whole shift of smokeeaters standing around watching every move you make. Not talking, but man, judging the hell out of you. They're pros and they have one thought in mind: "Can Junior here cut it? Is he going to panic and kill this dude because he's freaked out? Worse yet, if I go down in the street is he going to be able to pull me back from the brink?" Firefighters are judgmental bastards and they do not cut their own any slack, none, zero. The young fireman/paramedic knows this and knows he will just get frigging eviscerated if he makes one false move.

When he returned to the firehouse, it was quiet. He went into the bathroom and threw some cold water on his face. Studying his face in the mirror, he slowly exhaled. This was his moment. This was his internal review of his actions of the past few hours. There was no one else present. The house remained quiet. No celebrations. No fist pumps. This was what it felt like to be a pro. A quiet moment for a gut check. There was no bullshitting here. The reflection in the mirror was pensive, lost in thought, relieved more than anything else. "Did I do everything right? Did I perform to standard? Did I react quickly enough? Did I do make any mistakes? Did I do everything by the book? Did I improvise properly?

Check, check, check. Damn straight I did. We pulled that dude back from the brink of death and he goes home to fight another day. I did what I was trained to do. I did it fast and I did it in front of my boys without a second's hesitation. I performed to standard and tradition. Michael is going home to his family in a couple of days and he probably has had ankle sprains that hurt more and lasted longer."

A day of two later, the young fireman was sitting at home feeding the baby. She was a hot mess. Frigging split pea baby food everywhere except her mouth. The area around her high chair looked like a homeless shelter. She looks like some green alien from another dimension had slimed her.

The fireman's mind wandered off the task at hand. He was thinking about Mike, his performance, not so much about feeding Miss Godzilla.

He smiled, for at that moment he realized it was all good. At that moment, he knew it without question. He had the "Right Stuff".

"I can do this shit," he thought. "The hard work, the studying, the practical exams, the internships, it all came together and there were no lingering doubts. He was at this moment right where he should be. He was the total package and he had one more advantage that no other professionally trained paramedic in the world had.

He had the DNA of a *King*. He understood this. He embraced it. He had no choice. In some ways, it was a burden. He would always be held to a higher standard than his contemporaries. When he had blood pooling around his ankles and was elbow deep in guts, he knew he would always have this.

He, *Paramedic/Firefighter Matt Christian Zydlo*, son of Dr. Stanley M. Zydlo, Jr., M.D. was born for this life. He was right where he should be ---in the eye of the storm.

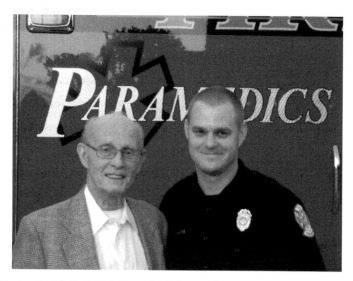

Dr. Stanley M. Zydlo Jr. M.D. and Schiller Firefighter/Paramedic Matt Zydlo.
Courtesy Matt Zydlo.

EPILOGUE

*"It is foolish and wrong to mourn the men
who died. Rather we should
thank God that such men lived."*
– *General George S. Patton*

Almost all the vestiges of youth were gone. In his eighth decade, Stan Zydlo had almost come full circle. Ninety-nine percent of today's paramedics have no idea who he was. He had outlived three children. He had buried dozens of colleagues, friends and family members. He was almost the "last man standing." Yet, yet the fire still raged. He read every medical journal he could lay his hands on. He was current on all the latest practices. He had not treated anyone in an emergency room in years, but if you were badly injured in a car accident, you would be very fortunate if Stan Zydlo happened to be in the area.

He still had it up until the end, almost. The "Right Stuff" had never deserted him. Mentally, he could still do it. Physically, not so much. Several open heart surgeries, three major heart attacks, a hip replacement, shoulder surgeries, some bad head injuries in falls. There were days when he was totally exhausted. He was just damn tired. Don't let anyone kid you. The grind of over fifty years of emergency room lifesaving medicine is unlike treating ulcers or skin conditions. ER medicine is dog year territory. Basically, for every year of snooze medicine, ER medicine equals seven years. A forty-year career is like 280 normal years. Think about the math for a moment.

I was in New Hampshire on Wednesday, June 3, 2015, when I received a text message from Matt Zydlo, Stan's son, the Paramedic/Fireman. It simply said, "*Dad has passed.*"

I wasn't surprised because Stan had been steadily declining for the last couple years. It was a long, drawn out, slow death. He had not been doing well for some time and all of us knew the end was in sight. Stan knew it. Frankly, it was a relief because he was sick, miserable and declining in every respect.

Getting a second chance in any endeavor is rare. Getting a second chance at life after a catastrophic medical event or accident was practically unheard of prior to 1972. Stan Zydlo just may have been the "King of second chances". On a least one occasion, his paramedics saved his life. There are now millions of people worldwide who have received a second chance thanks largely to Dr. Stan Zydlo and his paramedics.

At a luncheon of retired paramedics, a few months before he died, Dr. Zydlo showed up. It was akin to Eisenhower showing up for lunch at the officer's club. Everyone stopped talking and these old warhorses were, well, *excited*. They jumped up, shook his hand, man hugged, laughed. To a man, almost giddy that Dr. Zydlo had come to eat with them. The respect had not faded one bit. They all credit him with the success of their profession.

An interesting phenomenon with these guys is there total lack of self-importance. They are salt of the earth, middle class guys who collectively performed, heroically, thousands of time throughout the years. To a person, they will tell you, "Hey, we were Doc's eyes and hands. We only did what he taught us."

Though they were far more than "Doc's eyes and hands," they were the standard bearer for hundreds of thousands of future paramedics. They performed in every conceivable hardship and human condition. They were in the trenches with society's dirty little secrets, the drug overdoses, the homeless, the sick, the infirmed, the poor---every day, every moment, they performed in magnificent and creative ways. These originals are national treasures. They, along with Dr. Zydlo, are what helped make this country great. We owe them a collective debt we can never repay.

It was the twilight of Stan's existence and he knew it. The remaining fire chiefs and the original paramedics knew it. The conversations were a little forced; not much new to talk about. Many of the old guard have died or moved out of state. Their numbers are dwindling fast. In fifteen or twenty years, they may all be gone. But these men know exactly what they created. They were, collectively and individually, heroic in almost every professional endeavor they undertook.

Until now, none of them really considered what their contribution to society was. They don't think in those terms. Most of them are exactly like Dr. Zydlo in demeanor and attitude. They never sought the spotlight. They never went "Hollywood." They saved lives. They spread their gospel. They trained generations of paramedics and their paramedics trained subsequent paramedics. A system of excellence was born.

Today, one can become famous by having a fat ass or doing a sex tape with a famous boyfriend and "accidentally" leak it on the internet. These men---the fire chiefs and the "Zydlo-trained" paramedics--are responsible for saving tens of millions of lives, yet nobody knows who they are. Such is the state of America today.

So, how do we compare what Stan Zydlo did? In a sports analogy we would compare him to Babe Ruth, Jack Nicholas, Michael Jordan, Cal Ripken or Walter Payton. Those are nice comparisons, but there is no way to compare what Dr. Zydlo and the paramedic system accomplished. Hundreds of millions of lives were impacted. There is no way to legitimately measure the impact of this program in terms of human variables. How do we begin?

In medical terms, there are giants: Jonas Salk, the Mayo Brothers, Virginia Apgar, Michael E. DeBakey. These are the legends. Their names immediately jump out to even the least well read. Where does Stanley M. Zydlo stand among these giants of medicine? I would argue that he was the most important person in medicine in the last fifty years. He is peerless. No one, not one medical practitioner in the last century has been more responsible for saving lives than Stan Zydlo.

The Emergency Medical System in the modern world is the most cutting edge, incredibly efficient, medical apparatus known to man. On a daily basis, it saves thousands of lives. In the streets, your living room, at the park, at a construction site two hundred feet above ground level, paramedics save lives every minute of every day.

The system has become so commonplace, so routine, so inbred into our collective DNA that we don't give it a second thought. Nada. Nothing. We expect it. If you experience chest pains while waiting in your doctor's office, the paramedics will be called. How about that for irony? The fact that the entire medical community has so thoroughly embraced Dr. Zydlo's EMS is simply amazing considering the initial blowback from the same established medical community.

We just know if we get badly injured, if we have a cardiac episode, a stroke, diabetic shock, are in an airplane crash, have a drug overdose or gunshot wound that generally within six minutes there will be an incredibly well-trained, lifesaving machine rolling up to save our life. The machine's total existence, its whole being has one purpose and that is to keep us alive, get us to a hospital and all of the resources available there to save us.

What is almost never mentioned is the economic impact that Dr. Zydlo's little experiment has had. Have you looked at an emergency room bill lately? Do you have any idea what kind of bill gets generated when you are delivered to an emergency room via an ambulance? In Florida, during the years 2011 and 2012, the average bill was $8,342.00. Only six north Florida hospitals had an average charge under $1,000. This does not include the cost of the paramedics and ambulance.[38]

How many people go to the emergency room via ambulance? The number of non-injury ER visits in which chest pain was the primary reason was five million in 1999-2000 and five and a half million in 2007-2008, a difference that is not statistically significant. The percentage of ER visits for chest pain decreased ten percent during this time, from ten percent to nine percent.[39]

So, if you took five and half million visits to the ER via ambulance and the average bill for those five and a half million visits was $8,342.00, that means ER departments billed somewhere in the neighborhood of forty-five million dollars in one year just for cardiac-related visits. As Dr. Zydlo predicted from the beginning, this emergency medical system was a financial juggernaut of unknown riches. Add on cardiac surgery, hospital rooms, intensive care costs, meds, etc. and the cost benefit to the hospitals is in the trillions.

Would it be unfair to say that not only was Stan Zydlo indirectly responsible for the saving of millions of lives, but he also was responsible for the creation of the largest profit center in the history of medicine? I am guessing that, at some point, he wished he had copyrighted some of the program in the old days.

The human and economic impact attributable to Dr. Zydlo is mind boggling. There is simply no way to measure it. His contribution to medicine, the EMS and lastly, the economics, is something we are not likely to ever see again in medicine.

"I have fought a good fight. I have finished my course.
I have kept the faith."
(2 Timothy 4.7)

The funeral procession was three miles long. As we passed the fire-houses in multiple towns and cities in the northwest suburbs of Chicago, the on duty firemen stood outside at attention, saluting. It was heart wrenching.

I was okay at the wake. I was okay at the funeral mass. I was good when we carried Dr. Zydlo's casket through the Fire Department Honor Guard. It was hard, but I was okay with it all. The pageantry, the honor I felt from these public servants that Zydlo created, it just hung in the air like mustard gas. It was emotional and it was tearing the heart out of me, but I was still okay.

I was not okay when we passed our last firehouse and these young, good-looking firemen were all standing outside in duty shorts saluting, and brother you know they meant everything that salute meant which is the ultimate sign of respect between colleagues.

Then it happened---the ultimate moment in a lifetime of moments. As we approached a small strip mall (the kind you see everywhere in America), here was where all those feelings of loss fell on me like the proverbial avalanche.

At the corner of the strip mall on a little raised berm, stood three young Mexican guys. They were clearly just landscaping and working like you see about a million Mexicans a day doing in this country. These guys were not working at the moment. Standing at attention on the berm in their work clothes, they all had edge trimmers, rakes and what not in their left hands, but they stood with their right hands covering their hearts. Looking straight ahead and standing tall, they showed respect for a guy they had no idea in world who he was. But, I tell you this with all seriousness, this small act of respect just slayed me.

There was not a chance in hell they knew who was being transported to the cemetery. All they knew was that all these fire trucks, these ambulances, all these cars, meant that this funeral had to be for someone who was important, someone who was the shit, some hot stuff, bigger than life dude. It was at that moment that the loss hit me. My chest tightened up and my breath was gone. The moment I saw these three working guys standing there at attention, showing as much respect as they could to a total stranger was the moment I knew that this was permanent.

It really is the little things that count in life---The kind word, the friend who shows up and helps you carry an old couch out to the curb, the Mexican guys standing at attention as a funeral procession drives by. That was the moment that I knew Stan would just love. He would love the fact that these working men, (his favorite kind of people) would stop what they were doing and stand respectfully as a long train of a hundred vehicles or more slowly and deliberately passed by.

He would have appreciated the fire departments' efforts in sending him off. He would have enjoyed the newspaper articles, the public awareness of his death. But, man, he would have jumped up and cheered those three Mexican landscapers. That would have been the cherry on top the sundae for him.

Heroes do not get a pass on death. The end is the same for the village idiot as it is for a Congressional Medal of Honor recipient. Nobody leaves alive or unscarred. Today, with the exception of the military and first responders, heroes are in short supply. Today, we have Hipsters. We have an overdose of political correctness. Frankly, we have a mess of biblical proportions and someone like Dr. Stanley M. Zydlo could not accomplish anything close to what he accomplished for 1972 on. But the erosion of what Dr. Zydlo and that inaugural class of men started has begun. In death, Dr. Zydlo does not have to take on that fight and so, perhaps, it is fortunate that he will not have to gear up for a last confrontation.

Predictably, there will be criticism for writing about these heroes. There will be naysayers. There will be rebuttal articles about how many people are "killed by paramedics or ER docs". This is what occurs today. It comes with the territory. Stan Zydlo had seen it again and again. Remember, the "Para Gestapo Medic" cracks? Well, everything comes full circle and here we are.

The circle for Stan Zydlo is now closed. The mischievous twinkle in his eyes is gone. He is finally at rest. To the very end, he was still in search of how he could contribute. He was a giver to the bitter end.

Until the very end, he never listened to the critics. He didn't have time because as we all now know, Dr. Stanley M. Zydlo, Jr. was on a mission and you'd better get the hell out of his way or he would run right over you.

IN APPRECIATION

It has been my very special privilege and honor to write this book. My relationship with Stan Zydlo lasted more than twenty years. There is no question that my relationship with him was one of the great joys of my life. No project like this is done in a vacuum, especially a project whose scope covers forty-plus years. I did this for one reason and that was because of the immense respect and love I had for Stan Zydlo. His was a story that needed telling. He was an American hero with few peers. I have done everything in my power to tell his story frankly and honestly. It has been my very special privilege and honor to write this book. Any mistakes in this work are solely my responsibility and I apologize in advance to anyone I may have inadvertently forgotten to acknowledge.

My Kitchen Cabinet who always read this with a lot of enthusiasm and encouragement were always brilliant in their own crazy ways:

Liz Reed, my wife and all around brilliant trial attorney. In addition, she is a great woman of grace and compassion. Her support is always present. She is also my primary English teacher. She is always amazed at my total lack of a basic English education. Nevertheless, she gets me and she is able to make me look much brighter then I actually am.

Tom Wright. My Harvard-educated and brilliant Hollywood tactician who has great taste and a fifth sense about what works and does not work. Always honest and always kind, he is a true friend and corroborator

Pat Picarrelli , brilliant and talented author in his own right. Tough as nails former NYPD Lieutenant, Vietnam Vet, young at heart dude, who nursed me throughout the project.

Nick Massarella, Self-taught, self-made, brilliant businessman, my dear friend who always tells it like it is.

Grace Castle, my writing mentor and "work wife" for many years, whose patience with me shocked everyone. A brilliant editor and writer herself, she has always encouraged me and kept me centered.

The Zydlo children whose father was always proud of and who contributed greatly to this effort. *Matt Zydlo, Kate Zydlo* and *Brad Zydlo*.

The past and current *fire* chiefs who were always helpful and generous with their time and institutional knowledge.

A special thanks to Arlington Heights Retired Chief Bruce Rodewald and Rolling Meadows Retired Chief Ted Loesch, who has a hundred years of institutional knowledge between them. They always were available and helpful.

I would also like to thank the following individuals for their input and historical knowledge: NYPD Detective (Ret) John Baeza, Mt. Prospect Fire Chief Larry Pairitz, (Ret), Arlington Heights IL. Paramedic Bill Dressel, (Ret), Arlington Heights, IL. Battalion Fire Commander William H. Essling, Arlington Heights IL Fire Department Historian Charles Kramer, Mrs. Nancy Rodewald, Arlington Heights IL Fire Department Captain Jack Benson, (Ret)., Chicago Fire Department Deputy District Chief Jeffrey A. Lyle, Chicago Fire Department EMS Training Division Instructor Deborah Ford, CFD Medical Administrator Leslie Stein-Spencer, Palatine IL Fire Chief Scott Anderson, Melisa Fraase, Father Robert Mitchell, Arlington Heights IL Fire Department Paramedic Glenn Amundson, (Ret). Arlington Heights IL Fire Department Paramedic Dean Stewart, (Ret). Mrs. Nancy McKillop, Rolling Meadows IL Fire Chief Scott Franzgrote, Hoffman Estates Fire Chief Jeff Jorian, Glenview IL Fire Department Paramedic Brian Gaughan, (Ret), Gloria Siolidis, Jennie Siolidis, Firefighter Mike Bloom, Norman Morrill, Bryan Smith, Joe Halderman, Josephine Cozzi, CFD Paramedic Chief & author Marjorie Leigh Balbam, Aleka Lach,

Chicago Fire Dept. Lieutenant "Riv" Rivera, CFD Engineer Paul Strubbe, CFD Firefighter Dominic Mercado, CFD Firefighter/Paramedic Mark Kovacevich, CFD Tower 14 Captain "Billy" DiPinto, CFD Firefighter CFD Wally Obrochta, CFD Firefighter CFD Pat Fahrenbach, CFD Firefighter Chris Tolbert, and CFD Paramedic Field Chief Beth Ciolino.

Lastly, the men and woman who toil in the streets serving the public and who opened up their hearts and homes to me. There are many things in this world that are a mess. The fire service and paramedics are not. They are a gift and their overall contribution to society is mind boggling.

As I have finished this during the election season I have given a lot of thought as to how to improve our country and get it back on track and I believe that the solution is simple enough. All we have to do is vote in firemen and paramedics and let them run the country for a while. What do we have to lose? Does anyone who even has a moderate amount of intelligence still believe that the politicians who have been destroying this country slowly, but surely, deserve any further chances?

In all seriousness just consider this. Who do you call in an emergency? Who shows up tens of thousands of times a day in this country and almost always does a job that often reaches up into miracle territory? Day in and day, out the men and woman of our fire departments do, and they do it without any interference from their politicians. In fact, they largely keep them at bay and out of the lifesaving and fire business. That is, no doubt, a major factor in their continuing effectiveness.

Finally to you, *the reader* for being interested enough to pick this up and read it. It is my hope that you enjoyed this and learned something about the special human beings who created this program and continue to save our lives, in spite of our collective silliness and general ungratefulness.

– Paul Ciolino
Chicago, Illinois

POSTSCRIPT

The scene of a victim's worst day.

There is a good reason why the paramedics in a busy ambulance have a hard time staying on the job until they retire. Simply put it's the job. They are constantly, without exception, exposed and witness to the worst of human behavior. These are the men and woman who are the front line. They get it raw and unedited and always deal with the immediate aftermath of life's cruelties.

They are the people who see the little kids who catch the stray bullet while sleeping in their crib. They are the people who deal with a 17-year-old who just got shot four times because he had the wrong color sweater on. They are the people who hold the hands of a dying mother who is getting ready leave this life. Finally, they, better than almost anyone else in this life, get up every morning knowing they get to do this all over again.

They are every bit as human as the next person and yet the mental anguish they suffer is equal to their worst case scenario. They know what kind of pain you have and how bad it is. They deal with the shock and unbelievable pain of a parent who has just lost a child, the wife of a forty-year-old man who just had the big gripper, and the four dead kids scattered in the street after a drunk driver plowed into their family's van. They work every holiday and weekend. They have a front row seat to the war on drugs and its miserable failure.

They do this because they know that they are dealing with people who are for certain having the worst day of their life. In the last moments of someone's life they get to see that individual as they truly are. They, better than anyone else, understand just how precious and valuable a human life is. They also understand that taking life less than lightly is a huge mistake. They get it---and they *live* it.

They understand the high stakes poker game being played out in the street. They are sickened by it and yet they have no room left for that. The level of senseless violence that constantly swirls around them is never ending. They are the human garbage dumps, which is worse than a real dump because a real dump is eventually shut down. They don't have that luxury. They hate the carnage and the people who create it. They love the citizens who try to make the best of the situation.

When five Dallas Texas police officers were executed at a street protest, a Dallas Police Officer posted the following *Facebook* note the next day:

"Fire did not get enough credit, they were moving with us in ambulances toward Market Street, toward the gun fire. Every single time we told them to get out of the shooting zone the driver would just keep yelling, "Just tell us where they are," referring to our downed officers who had been shot."

"Toward the gun fire" is the key phrase here. They are not armed. Ninety-nine percent of them do not wear bulletproof vests. Yet, unlike any other job outside of law enforcement, they go willingly toward the gunfire, the riot, the burning building, and any other active disaster that you can conjure up. They do it because as Dr. Zydlo said, "People need help when they need it".

This is worth remembering because they don't get a vote as to what they witness. The next time you see an ambulance, please remember this and remember that it happens every day in every part of the country.

You might also want to remember that a guy named *Stanley M. Zydlo, Jr.* was the person most responsible for this.

ENDNOTES

1. "The Merciful Magic of Ether-Anesthetics in the Civil War" A.J Wright, Anesthesiology News, March 2013, Volume 39:3

2. Six degrees of separation is the theory that everyone and everything is six or few steps away, by way of introduction, from any other.

3. Job, Macarthur (1996).*Air Disaster– Volume 2.* Weston Creek: Aerospace Publications. pp.47–60.ISBN1875671196

4. Chicago Firefighters Union Local 2 website. From the history section.

5. From the internet and "Find a Grave" website at http://www.finda-grave.com

6. Chicago Department of Aviation, O'Hare history section at www.flychicago.

7. Ted Seals, Chicago Sun-Times article 12/7/75

8. Jose Santiago (The Current Fire Commissioner for The CFD) Chicago Area Fire website blog, dtd 02/22/15

9. Firefighters Local Union Two website. CFD History page.

10. NBC News, Illinois has long legacy of Public Corruption. 12/09/08

11. From WNEZ 91.5 radio stations. By; Tricia Bobada, 11/5/12

12. Wikipedia

13. City of Chicago data portal.

14. Naloxone, also known asNarcanamong other names, is a medication used to reverse the effects of opioids especially inoverdose. Naloxone may be combined within the same pill as an opioid to decrease the risk of misuse. When given intravenously it works within two minutes.

15. Synthetic cannabis(synthetic marijuana), or technicallysynthetic cannabinoid receptor agonists aredesigner drugsthat mimic the effects of cannabis sprayed onto an herbal base material. Wikipedia.

16. Anelectrocardiogram (EKG or ECG) is a test that checks for problems with theelectrical activity of your heart. An EKG shows theheart's electrical activity as line tracings on paper. Web MD, date unknown

17. Wildman is a fictitious name.

18. Pancreatitis is a condition that may be mild and self-limiting, though it can also lead to severe complications that can be life threatening. The acute person in the world, so that a chain of "a friend of a friend' statements can be made to connect any two people in a maximum of six steps. It was *originally* set out by Frigyes Karinthy in 1929. Wikipedia

19. Fivethirtyeight.com article by Mona Chalabi, DTD: 3/19/15

20. Hannibal's elephant's name was Surus. New York Times article, THE MYSTERY OF HANNIBAL'S ELEPHANTS. John Noble Wilford, Published: September 18, 1984

21. The Paramedics by James O. Page, Backdraft Publications, Morristown New Jersey.

22. CrossFit is a strength and conditioning program consisting mainly of a mix of aerobic exercise, calisthenics (body weight exercises), and Olympic weight lifting.[15]CrossFit Inc. describes its strength and conditioning program as "constantly varied functional movements

executed at high intensity across broad time and modal domains,"[16] with the stated goal of improving fitness, which it defines as "work capacity across broad time and modal domains." Wikipedia.

23. Internet, From Wikipedia page titled "Emergency"

24. Internet, From Wikipedia page titled "American Airlines Flight 191"

25. Form of pancreatitis, in its most severe form, can have deleterious effects on many other body organs, including the lungs and kidneys.

26. Don Giovanni, in full The Libertine Punished; or, Don Giovanni, Italian II dissolute punito; ossia, il Don Giovanni, opera in two acts by Wolfgang Amadeus Mozart (Italian libretto by Lorenzo da Ponte) that premiered at the original National Theatre in Prague on October 29, 1789.

27. Almost every artery in the body branches off of the aorta. These arteries supply blood to the brain, other vital organs liver stomach, small andlarge bowel,spinal cord and nerves, bones, muscles, and cells that allow the body to function.

28. Almost every artery in the body branches off of the aorta. These arteries supply blood to the brain, other vital organs liver stomach, small andlarge bowel,spinal cord and nerves, bones, muscles, and cells that allow the body to function.

29. Elizabeth Rosenthal New York Times Magazine, Paying til it hurts E.R. Part 5 12/02/13

30. By Andrew Fegelman, Chicago Tribune Staff Writer, February 24, 1994

31. Financial numbers drawn from a combination of internet sources

32. Sarak Kliff, An average ER visit costs more than an average month's rent. The Washington Post. 03/02/13

33. Lawyers and settlements.com, author unknown, dtd 05/08/15

34. James Hirby, The Law Dictionary, internet article, (date unknown)

35. The Merna Law Group, Merna law.com, Author and date unknown.

36. The cost-benefit-analysis (CBA) is also defined as a systematic process for calculating and comparing benefits and costs of a project, decision or government policy. Wikipedia. (2015)

37. Yanki Tauber, Chad.com internet article. Date unknown

38. Chicago Tribune, Ameet Sachdev, 02/18/16

39. Researchers Tool from FloridaHealthFinder.gov

40. Bhuiya F, Pitts SR, McCaig LF. Emergency department visits for chest pain and abdominal pain: United States, 1999-2008. NCHS data brief, No 43. Hyattsville, MD: National Center for Health Statistics. 2010.

AUTHOR'S NOTE

I have never written a biography. Never once thought of it and frankly taking on such a complex and historically important subject, as this is it has simply been overwhelming at times throughout this journey. I was Stan Zydlo's friend for over twenty years. I saw him at the height of his powers and I saw him at his worst moments. I stood with him and his wife Joyce as they buried two of their children, something no parent should have to experience. I was there for Stan's physical decline, which was frankly devastating to watch.

However, old age is God's way of letting us know how human and weak we are. It is the ultimate great equalizer that predicts our forthcoming demise. Stan being the intellectual giant he was, recognized this long before it really took hold and slowly destroyed him. He did not go easily. He scraped, clawed, and did everything humanly possible to stay relevant and useful. He was well into his seventies before any serious decline happened. The body caved before the brain did. Multiple heart attacks, multiple open heart surgeries, hip replacements, shoulder surgeries, he became the ultimate ER patient "visiting" frequently.

In a way, it was funny in that dark humor funny manner because when Stan hit that ER he still thought he was in charge of the ER. He wasn't so much a patient as he was a walking, talking legend that still felt he had the "right stuff". The respect that he was always shown was admirable.

He was of course all that and more. The Docs knew it, the nurses knew it and anyone within earshot knew it. Stan was diagnosing and considering the cause of action while it was happening. He had this amazing ability to step outside of the pain or swirling hurricane engulfing him and look at it as a professional and not as a patient. Despite any pain or discomfort, he was in charge and he would take his last breath knowing this.

Like all true leaders Stan had his detractors. There was a whole class of people who were silently hoping he would fall on his ass. There were people who actively campaigned against him and backstabbed him at every opportunity---other doctors, the nurses, and hospital administrators, the list was daunting. Most people can easily be baited into long drawn out, in-house political fights, and mini wars, over this sort of behavior. Not Zydlo. He saw it and he knew what was afoot.

He was tempted just because of his combative nature. But, he never bit. He always kept his eye on the prize. In his mind his paramedics and patients came first and everything else was background noise.

That was his genius and just remarkable self-discipline kicking in. It sounds simple, but it is not. Zydlo knew human nature and he understood it like few people did.

He was the ultimate chess player and consistently way ahead of 99% of the population. Age, maturity, and experience do that. Throw in a healthy dose of genius IQ and you are simply unstoppable. He was a force for over forty-five years and only injuries, illness, and age was able to finally slow him down.

Retired Rolling Meadows Fire Chief and inaugural paramedic Ted Loesch described Zydlo best when he said, "Stan was abrupt, he was rude, and he had a bad reputation in some circles. He was also intense and determined. He suffered no fools and he would make no concessions." These things made him the best of the best and without him none of this would have happened for years to come.

There was also the secret weapon in the person of Joyce Zydlo. The unsung hero in this drama was Joyce. Most women in her position would not have tolerated their husband's laser beam attention to the emergencies, and seemingly endless interruption of missed birthdays, anniversaries, and other significant family events. How about an emergency services radio blasting in your bedroom night after night, in fact year after year, with tragedy and death blasting you out of a sound sleep?

They never ever got through a meal in restaurant without Stan being called out to an emergency. Joyce frequently took a cab home with the kids in tow. Some restaurants would just bring a doggy bag at the beginning of a meal knowing that Stan would never make it through the whole meal. On one occasion, he was called and he discovered halfway out the door that the emergency was in the ladies room in the restaurant he was running out of. How about every romantic moment being interrupted with the EMS radio blasting "Hey Doc, we need you here, right now!"

Not many spouses of either sex would tolerate that year in and year out. Joyce did it with a smile and the knowledge that this was who she married. For better and worse meant something to her and although not much thought has ever been given to what Joyce had to do to support Stan and make this all happen, none of this would have happened without her support and love. Stan knew. Anyone who ever saw them together knew exactly what her worth was to this whole paramedic business.

Joyce Zydlo is every bit as responsible for the early success of the program as anyone. Had she insisted that her husband "have a normal medical practice" the paramedic profession would have been set back several years and consequently a few more hundred thousand lives would have been lost.

So, if we were to start handing out medals of valor to people for their role in this real life drama, Joyce Zydlo would be high up on the list to receive one.

Stan's youngest four children also played a part. All of them Josh, (now deceased) Matt a fireman and paramedic in Schiller Park, IL. Kate a schoolteacher, and Brad an operations foreman with an international retail giant, suffered along with their mother. They were primarily the victims of Stan's success. They were the ones who grew up with mostly a view of their father's narrow ass running out the front door to one disaster or another.

They are all amazing, well balanced, bright, and successful. I have never heard them whisper one bad word about their father. They grew up in emergency rooms and firehouses. They knew "the family business". They understood exactly who their father was and they worshiped him, as he did them. They also had a remarkable way of letting Stan know that this "hero shit" didn't cut it at home. I have seen the kids just light him up at times and Stan actually liked it. His pride in his family was always evident and he knew that it grounded him and made him a better human being.

Finally, there are the paramedics and especially that inaugural group of 107 who hit the street on December 1, 1972. Those 107 men are the collective founders of the paramedic service. All subsequent EMTs and Paramedic's owe their livelihood and professional status to those men for the very simple fact that they trail blazed this entire profession and the success or failure of their initial work allowed what was to become the single biggest lifesaving mechanism in the modern world.

I have met many of the 107. Most of them are old, some very old. Many of them have died. Here is what I can tell you about these men. They were all exceptionally bright. None of them, with the exception of Mt. Prospect firemen Ken Koeppen and Lowell Fell, had any formal medical training. They were all Caucasian and most of them had some military service. There were no women in the first several classes.

Most of them were, and still are, in long-term marriages. They are stable and responsible human beings who more often than not, put everyone else's wellbeing and comfort ahead of their own. They do what men were once taught as being paramount, they take care of their fellow man.

They were the type of men who made this country the greatest country in human history. Their backs are what carried the heavy load of this program in the early days and the reality of the situation is that very few people in their profession never mind society will ever know just what a giant almost unequaled achievement this was.

They are now just your typical older seniors. They are deep into the fourth quarter of their life and they are no longer actively out there saving lives and having incredible doses of adrenaline coursing through their veins. Well, maybe retired paramedic Eddie Kemper does, but any time the rest of them spend in an Emergency Room is generally because of their own medical issues.

There have been, since that day in December of 1972, at least one million of these professionals plying this trade and trolling in the trenches. They single handily changed the face of emergency medicine and prehospital care. They are responsible for the saving of tens of millions of lives and they have done it quietly, professionally, and without too much self-promotion. If they were Navy Seals, this would have been about the 100th book about them. Actually, it's the first and that should clue you into just how humble they remain.

One of my greatest joys in writing this book has been getting to know these men and woman who came later on a personal level. Collectively, I have, outside of the military, never met a nicer or a more humble group of professionals. They are terribly underpaid and hugely underappreciated, or at least until they are hammering the paddles to your chest to shock you back to life. You become a fan pretty quick then.

They can take it and they can dish it out with the best of them. On one occasion, in the early days, a Rolling Meadows IL paramedic was having a hard time getting an IV needle in the correct vein. Zydlo was in the hospital on the radio listening to the drama unfold. He was not happy. He was tapping his foot like Max Weinberg on the drums and his blood pressure rose by the second. After a few minutes, he couldn't stand it anymore, so he grabbed the radio mike and says, "If you don't get that needle in the right vein, right now, I will stick it in your dorsal vein in your penis when you get here." The correct vein was immediately located and the paramedic stayed out of Stan's gun sights for the next several days.

I was also very fortunate to meet and observe many firemen during this project and in addition to being hospitable and friendly, they were also open and honest about the day to day stuff that they are witness to. Everybody was about as helpful as they could be and I will remain eternally grateful for their generosity and frankness.

The paramedics regularly get abused by their own departments and frankly the treatment they receive in most emergency rooms borders on scandalous. In spite of these very real issues, they constantly perform above and beyond the call of duty and they do it for all the right reasons. Their basic DNA requires this. Forty-plus years of heroic and incredible service to the community is now collectively hardwired into them. They self-police. They are their own harshest critics. There are very few professions that operate this cleanly or effectively.

Finally, for those of you who bought this book and thinking that you are about to read something like, "*Quantum Field theory in Curved Spacetime and Black Hole Thermodynamics*", please be advised to return this immediately and get your money back. This book is about working men and woman who live and work in the street. At times it is profane and it is real. To chronicle it any other way would be a disservice to the men and women it is about.

I am hopeful that this book honors Stan and the paramedics. Their accomplishments and historical significance were a pleasure to chronicle. I apologize in advance for not telling all of their unique stories. To a man, they all played a significant, historical role, along with their wives and children who suffered equally in those early years. I leave it up to the reader to judge their place in history.